Hauke Fürstenwerth

Ouabain

Hauke Fürstenwerth

Ouabain

a gift from paradise

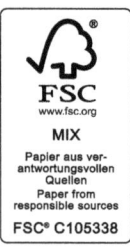

Bibliographic information of the German National Library:
The German National Library lists this publication in the German National Bibliography; detailed bibliographical data is available on the Internet at http://dnb.dnb.de

2018 Hauke Fürstenwerth

Images:
Wikimedia: Edgar 181 (18, 19, 20), Klaus Hoffmeier (19, 20), Jakov (55), Sven Drefahl (187), American Heart Association (103), Time Inc. (104), SPIEGEL Verlag (106),
all other images: Hauke Fürstenwerth

Production and publishing:
BoD - Books on Demand, Norderstedt
ISBN: 978-3-7481-6576-7

acknowledgement

I would like to thank Dr. Waltraud Kern-Benz, Stuttgart, for providing me with extensive documents on the work of Dr. Berthold Kern.

Table of Contents

preamble

Ouabain is a natural substance that occurs in African lianas of the genus Strophanthus and in the shrub Acokanthera ouabaio, also native to Africa. Its chemical structure is similar to that of digitalis glycosides. Like the digitalis glycosides digoxin and digitoxin, ouabain has been used to treat heart disease. For the locals in Africa, Strophanthus was poison and remedy in one. In the mythology of the tribe of the Wilé in Upper Volta, this plant was sent from paradise to the earth to heal or punish people according to their merit. Ouabain (known as g-Strophanthin in German literature) has polarized the medical profession like hardly any other drug. Euphoric praise and devastating criticism characterised an extremely polemical and emotional dispute. *"The time will come, in which failure to timely start ouabain therapy will be condemned as medical malpractice."* With this prophecy the internist Ernst Edens (1876 - 1944), who held a chair at the University of Dusseldorf, in 1943 summarized his experiences with the cardiac glycoside ouabain. In 1985, the Munich cardiologist Erland Erdmann stated: *"there is no longer a reliable indication for ouabain, whether orally, perlingually or intravenously.* What was the reason for this change of mind? From which new findings could Erdmann derive his assessment? There were no studies in which ouabain had been compared with new drugs and proven to be inferior. Erdmann's assessment marked the end of a scientific debate in medicine that had been fiercely fought out over decades.

This book describes the eventful history of the heart medication oua-bain. The rise and fall of ouabain have already been described several times. Nearly all of the previous presentations concentrate on a public debate in the 1960s and 1970s on the causes of heart attacks between the Stuttgart-based internist Berthold Kern and the Heidelberg phar-macologist Gotthard Schettler. This dispute was not only debated in scientific journals, but also publicly in daily newspapers, magazines, radio and television reports. An objective, fact-based analysis of the history of ouabain is still lacking. I would like to close this gap with this book. This book is also meant to popularize the history of oua-bain in the Anglo-Saxon-world. Although ouabain still is the subject of intensive research, its use as a medicine is hardly known in Eng-lish-speaking countries. Although, even as early as 1948, Sir John McMichael, a pioneer in the field of cardiology in Britain, observed the advantageous qualities of the Strophanthus glycosides compared to digoxin and acknowledged *"We must also plead guilty to neglect of the study of the actions of the strophanthins ... ."* ouabain hardly has been used in the Anglo-Saxon-world [McMichael 1948].

Today, only a few older physicians remember this heart medication, which was once so popular in Europe and especially in Germany. Younger doctors don't know ouabain anymore. Textbooks mention it, if at all, only as a historical side note. Ouabain-based preparations are only available as over-the-counter homeopathic products or as *Defek-turarzneimittel[1]* that require a prescription. Is there more than just a historical interest in dealing with this "old" drug at all?

Two findings indicate that a reassessment of ouabain in the treatment of heart failure is also appropriate for scientific reasons. On the one hand, there is an urgent need for effective means of treating heart failure. Heart failure is the only disease whose incidence and preva-lence are steadily increasing in many developed countries. Despite

---

[1] Defekturarzneimittel are drugs that are manufactured in pharmacies in quantities of up to one hundred ready-to-deliver packages per day without the need for a manufacturing permit or drug approval according to the German Medicines Act.

modern treatment with beta-blockade and full angiotensin II modulation, the five-year mortality rate of heart failure is over 50% and corresponds to that of cancer. The efficacy of today's standard medication for the treatment of heart failure in absolute terms is only a few percentage points better than placebo. On the other hand, current research results show that ouabain has previously unknown therapeutic qualities which justify subjecting this drug to clinical re-evaluation.

Also in the current research on ouabain, qualities of ouabain are fiercely disputed. Like in the past, the dispute on ouabain again is dominated by hubris and personal vanity. A group of scientists is convinced that ouabain is an endogenous hormone. It is asserted that ouabain not only is a key factor in the pathogenesis of hypertension and heart failure but has significant implications in the pathogenesis of many common diseases, including renal failure, essential hypertension and heart failure.

These assertions are in stark contrast to decades of positive clinical experiences with ouabain in the treatment of heart diseases. In fact, recent research results confirm the cardio-protective effect of ouabain. In samples of human plasma that contained considerable levels of "endogenous ouabain" as detected by radioimmunoassay, with highly sensitive analytical methods no ouabain could be detected. These results confirm: there is no endogenous ouabain in human plasma. Thus the hypothesis of endogenous ouabain is refuted.

To understand the rise and fall of ouabain, one has to deal with the scientific basis of this drug, which has been uncovered in centuries of research, as well as with the findings on the causes of heart diseases. Scientific findings are not timelessly and irrevocably valid laws. They are subject to various influences and changes that can only be understood in a historical context.

Generations of researchers and physicians have shaped the history of ouabain. Outstanding personalities have developed fundamental findings that build on each other and have put them into clinical practice. The history of ouabain is also embedded in the development of the pharmaceutical industry and in the changes in the scientific disciplines on which it is founded. Pharmacology, genetics, molecular biology and other scientific disciplines have replaced clinical observations at the bedside as the starting point for the development of new drugs. Today, patients are treated with medication even without symptoms. The statistical risk for a probable disease has been established as an independent clinical manifestation. Guideline values for blood pressure, cholesterol and blood sugar define diseases. This change is also part of ouabain's history. The history of this cardiac glycoside is also marked by failures, false generalisations, ingenious intuition, polemical criticism, academic vanity, material interests and personal profit-seeking.

The story of ouabain is not over. Ouabain is still the subject of intensive basic research. Current research results enable a new interpretation of many years of therapeutic experience. These new findings - also in the context of current findings on the pathogenesis of heart diseases - show that this cardiac glycoside has untapped therapeutic potential. It is a matter of the heart of this book to illustrate this potential and hopefully to contribute to efforts to re-assess ouabain's therapeutic qualities fort he benefit of patients.

The history of ouabain is almost exclusively documented in German literature. In this book I make use of many original citations and literal quotations. For a better understanding I have translated these quotations into English. If some of the quotations appear to be incomprehensible, it is exclusively due to my translation and not to the original text.

Hauke Fürstenwerth

William Withering and the Red Foxglove

Plants and herbs have been used in all epochs of human history to produce remedies. Therapeutic experiences with plants and plant extracts have always been collected and described. The oldest traditional recipe collection for herbal remedies is more than 5,000 years old. It comes from Mesopotamia, the land between Euphrates and Tigris. Egyptian records for the use of medicinal plants date back to around 1,500 BC. Chinese records date back to 1,100 BC. In India, descriptions of the use of medicinal plants in the context of Ayurvedic medicine have already emerged around 1,000 BC. In the Middle Ages it was mainly the monasteries that preserved, documented and practiced the traditional knowledge about the use of medicinal plants. With the invention of letterpress printing in the 16th century, the knowledge of the healing power of plants was then laid down in the form of herbal books and thus made generally available. In the 18th century, scientists began to investigate the effects of medicinal plants in a targeted manner. Initially, the aim was to clarify which medicinal plant works best for which disease. In later centuries the investigations were extended to the pure ingredients contained in the medicinal plants, the elucidation of their chemical structure and their pharmacological effects. Towards the end of the 19th century, the chemical modification of the active ingredients was added. Many of the drugs used today are variations of natural substances found in plants.

One of the first systematic studies of the effects of a medicinal plant, the Red Foxglove (Digitalis purpurea), comes from the English physician William Withering. In 1785 he published the results of his studies under the title "*An Account of the Foxglove and some of its Medical Uses: with Practical Remarks on Dropsy and other Diseases*". Only one year later a German and a French translation were published. Interest in Withering's results also was expressed in America.

Since the Red Foxglove is not found in America, Withering supplied his American colleague Hall Jackson with seeds of the plant. Jackson cultivated the Red Foxglove and introduced Digitalis therapy of dropsy with Foxglove in America [Skou 1986].

Withering (1741 - 1799) studied medicine, botany and mineralogy at the University of Edinburgh. In 1766 he began his professional career as a clinician in a practice in Stafford, County Staffordshire. In 1775 Withering and his colleague John Ash took over a practice in Birmingham. In 1779 he was appointed to the medical team of the General Hospital in Birmingham, where he worked until his retirement in 1792. In addition, he continued his flourishing private practice.

Shortly before moving to Birmingham, Withering became aware of a herbal mixture for the treatment of dropsy (an abnormal accumulation of body fluids). The recipe for the mixture came from an old woman in Shropshire County. It also achieved healing successes in patients for whom treatment by doctors had failed. The healer's herbal mixture contained more than 20 different herbs. Withering, who also was trained as a botanist, writes that *"it was not very difficult for one conversant in these subjects, to perceive that the active herbs could be no other than Foxglove"*. Withering's decision to investigate the effect of Foxglove was reinforced by the experience of his colleague Dr. Cawley from Oxford, who suffered from an incurable water retention in his chest (hydrops pectoris) and could be cured by taking Foxglove roots [Skou 1986].

The Foxglove belongs to the plant genus of the plantain family (Plantaginaceae). There are about 25 species, which are native to Europe, North Africa and Western Asia. Of medical importance are the Red Foxglove (Digitalis purpurea) and the woolly Foxglove (Digitalis lanata). The use of Foxglove as a medicinal plant was first mentioned in a Valaisan herbal book in 1250 under the name "foxes glofa". In his book "Historia Stirpium" published in 1542, the German botanist and physician Leonhard Fuchs describes various Foxglove species in detail and gives them the name *Digitalis* [Greef 1981].

A Digitalis ointment and Digitalis tablets are mentioned 1650 for the first time in the official English list of medicines "Pharmacopeia Londoniensis". In 1748, the French doctor Francois Salerne describes the extreme toxicity of Gigitalis plants when fed to turkeys and urges caution when using these plants. When Withering began his Foxglove studies, this plant species was already an official part of several drug lists: 1744 Edinburgh Pharmacopeia, 1748 Paris Pharmacopeia, 1771 Wittenberg Pharmacopeia. Foxglove was recommended for the treatment of a wide range of diseases. Wound healing, headaches, asthma, rheumatism, and convulsions were only some of many diseases for which Foxglove preparations were used.

Withering knew from the healer's accounts from Shropshire County that the Foxglove has strong diuretic effects, often accompanied by severe vomiting and diarrhoea. He also knew about the extreme toxicity of the Foxglove. Accordingly carefully he planned his experiments. In the introduction to his book *Account of the Foxglove*, Withering lists four possibilities which he considered suitable for investigating the effects of the Foxglove. The investigations could be carried out chemically. At Withering's time, however, this method was limited to burning the substance and had proved useless until then. As a second possibility he saw the observation of Foxglove effects on animals. There were few reliable observations about the effects of medicinal herbs on animals and their significance for the effects on humans. Withering also rejected this method. For the same reason, he dispensed with a possible third alternative, the comparison with medicinal plants with similar effects. As the only reliable way to study the effects of the Foxglove, he chose the empirical use and observation of the effects on patients. Today we know that Digitalis has little effect on healthy humans and animals. If Withering had decided to study animals, he would not have found the effect of Digitalis. He was only able to study these in sick patients.

Such experiments in humans cannot be justified under current ethical standards. But it is not appropriate to judge Withering's actions by today's standards on the basis of today's knowledge. In the 18th century it was still common practice in many regions of Europe to burn women as witches for trivial reasons on the pyres. Withering's actions can only be judged in the cultural-historical context of his time and against the background of the knowledge available to him. At Withering's time there was no knowledge of the causes of the diseases to be treated, nor was it known how and why medicinal herbs and other remedies unfold their effects. The scientific disciplines of pharmacology and toxicology did not yet exist. William Withering's great merit is to replace the previously customary procedure of "trial and error" with a systematic approach and thus to open up new healing possibilities. It was not until 200 years after Withering's work on the Red Foxglove that drug laws were passed that today require extensive preclinical studies to be carried out before new drugs can be tested on humans.

Dr. Small, one of Withering's predecessors at the General Hospital in Birmingham, had arranged for one hour a day of free treatment for the destitute at the General Hospital. Withering continued this tradition. In this way, two to three thousand poor patients were treated each year. Withering selected suitable patients for his Foxglove studies from this patient pool. From 1776 to 1785 Withering treated 163 patients with different Foxglove preparations in graduated doses [Skou 1986].

The first task was to find a suitable dosage form for the Foxglove. Which parts of the plant are particularly suitable? How do they need to be prepared? In what dosage should they be administered? Powdered, dried leaves, which had been collected during the flowering period of the Foxglove, proved to be particularly suitable and effective. Aqueous extracts were only weakly effective, alcoholic extracts had too strong side effects. Withering observed such side effects even after the dried leaves were administered, but tried to exclude them to a large extent by reducing the dose. As optimal dosage Withering describes to administer Digitalis until side effects occur: *"let it be given 1-3 graine two times per day (65 - 200* mg*) of powder of the digitalis leaves ... and let it be continued till it either acts on the kid-*

neys, the stomach, the pulse or the bowles; let it be stopped upon the first appearance of any one of these effects". To suppress the side effects - especially nausea and vomiting - he recommended the simultaneous administration of opium [Somberg 1985].

In his experiments Withering found the extreme toxicity of the Foxglove confirmed. As toxic effects he lists: *"Illness, vomiting, diarrhoea, dizziness, visual disturbances, objects appear green and yellow; increased secretion of urine, slow pulse, down to 35 beats in a minute, cold sweat, cramps, fainting, death."* These effects occurred mainly at the high doses with which Withering began his investigations. *"I administered it in much too high doses over a much too long period of time."* Deaths were the result.

According to Withering's observations, Digitalis primarily acts as a diuretic, which was superior to all other diuretics known to date in the treatment of water retention in tissue. Withering also mentions the effect of Foxglove on cardiac activity: Digitalis has *"a power over the motion of the heart to a degree yet unobserved in any other medicine, and that this power may be converted to salutary ends."* At Withering's time, the causes of dropsy were not yet known. The realization that water retention is a consequence of heart failure only became established towards the end of the 19th century. Therefore, Withering did not attach any particular importance to the effect of Digitalis on the heart. The discovery that Digitalis is a potent means of treating heart disease has been reserved for later generations of physicians and scientists. Nevertheless, William Withering is regarded today as the father of Digitalis therapy. His studies of the Red Foxglove are a prime example of systematic studies that have ushered in a new era in medical research. The physician and Digitalis expert Albert Fraenkel (1864-1938) formulated in 1936: *"Withering's feat was that of an intuitive pharmacological-clinical concept. The use of Digitalis is not his glory title. He owes his immortality to the searching and finite finding of the correct dosage even today and the recognition and scheduled use of the pulse frequency as an indicator of the application and success of the therapy."* In recognition of his scientific achievements, William Withering was admitted to the Royal Society in London in 1785, the society with the greatest social prestige in 18th century England.

Withering's work on the effects of the Red Foxglove met with great interest among physicians, not only in England, but also in France and Germany. But the success was of limited duration. Although Withering gave precise instructions in the *Account of the Foxglove* on collecting Foxglove leaves - location of the plant, time of collection, storage method and more - many Digitalis preparations were of dubious and varying quality. Digitalis was used as a panacea against many diseases for which no effect could be achieved. The doses used were too high. Poisoning due to overdose was the rule. Until the late 19th century, Digitalis remained a controversial remedy with limited acceptance among doctors. This only changed when the causes of dropsy were recognized and advances in chemistry and pharmacology made it possible to isolate the active ingredients contained in Digitalis plants and study their pharmacological properties.

From arrow poison to medicine

The Strophanthus and Acokanthera species, which are native to Africa and parts of Asia, contain cardiac glycosides that are structurally similar to those of the Digitalis species. The glycosides serve the plants as a defense against predators. Humans and animals have also taken advantage of the toxicity of these plants. The African crested rat (*Lophiomys imhausi*) uses it for an extraordinary defense strategy. It chews the bark of highly toxic acokanthera shrubs, which contain the cardio-active glycoside g-Strophanthin (ouabain), and then applies the toxic saliva to the hair of its prominent crest. The sponge-like structure of the hair secures the saturation of the coat with poison loaded saliva by capillary forces. Dogs that attack the crested rat and come into contact with the poisonous coat show severe poisoning symptoms that can lead to death [Kingdon 2012]. Rats themselves are much less sensitive to steroid glycosides than other species. That's why the Acokanthera poison has no effect on them.

Many tribes in Africa have used preparations of Strophanthus and Acokanthera plants as arrow poisons. These were used both on the hunt for wild animals and in acts of war. Even large animals like elephants could be killed with the highly poisonous arrows. Poison arrows were important weapons in the arsenal of the African population in resisting invaders, slave hunters and colonial masters. In the British colonies the natives were forbidden to produce and possess arrow poisons and were threatened with drastic punishments. Even the cultivation of Strophanthus plants and the collection of Strophanthus seeds was punishable [Osseo-Asare 2014]. The recipes for the preparation of the poison mixtures were passed on as secret recipes only within the own tribe. Outsiders were not told which parts of the plant had to be harvested at what time and how they had to be processed and often enriched with other ingredients such as snake or scorpion poison.

African healers knew the medical value of Strophanthus plants very early on. Alcoholic extracts were produced by soaking the plant roots with subsequent fermentation. The bitter-tasting solutions were administered in small sips over a period of days or weeks. To avoid poisoning, the amount administered was carefully dosed by the healer. Muscle pain, open wounds, constipation, food poisoning, sexual diseases and heart disease were treated [Osseo-Asare 2014]. To the locals, Strophanthus was poison and remedy in one. In the mythology of the Wilé tribe in Upper Volta, this plant was sent from paradise to earth to heal or punish people according to their merit [Leuenberger 1972].

In the report of his expedition to Mozambique, during which he explored the Zambezi tributaries from 1857 to 1863, the Scottish missionary David Livingstone describes a poison that was used by the local warriors in the Shire highlands on Lake Najasasee to kill people and referred to as kombé. *"If you touch a tiny piece of this poison with your tongue, it is paralyzed."* Livingstone was accompanied on his expedition by the botanist John Kirk. His task was to look for plants that seemed suitable and profitable for commercial products. Kirk reports that a single poisoned arrow was enough to kill a buffalo, but the hunters often had to stay on the wounded animal's heels for half a day before the deadly effect occurred. Kirk kept some examples of the kombé poison arrows in a bag, in which he also kept his toothbrush. When he used it one morning in March 1859, he noticed a bitter taste. Kirk's pulse was elevated due to a feverish cold, but decreased significantly after using the toothbrush. Kirk attributed this rapid effect to a contamination of his toothbrush with the kombé poison. Kirk sent samples of the poison and parts of the plant from which the kombé poison was prepared to the Royal Botanical Institute in London (Kew Gardens). There the plant was first identified as Strophanthus hispidus, later correctly as Strophanthus kombé.

Several researchers have rendered outstanding services in the clarification of the active substance contained in Strophanthus kombé and its pharmacological properties. Thomas Richard Fraser (1841 - 1922)

- who taught pharmacognosy, pharmacy, pharmacology and therapy at the same time in Edinburgh - dealt most intensively with the kombé poison. He succeeded in isolating the pure active ingredient and characterised it as a glycoside. He was also able to show that the Strophanthus active ingredient has a pronounced cardiac effect and is suitable for therapy in humans. In 1885 Fraser reported on his first experiences with a Strophanthus tincture in patients and recommended its use in all forms of *cardiac fatigue* and as a diuretic. Fraser's work today is regarded as the basis for the application of Strophanthin to humans.

At the end of the 19th century, Digitalis preparations were a controversial remedy with limited acceptance by doctors due to their uncertain effects and their dreaded toxicity. Fraser's work nurtured the hope that Strophanthus glycosides might be a suitable replacement for Digitalis preparations. The Strophanthus research that began after 1885 was correspondingly intensive. As early as 1890, the number of scientific publications totalled more than one hundred. Intensive research has also been carried out in France and Germany on Strophanthus active ingredients.

French researchers in particular differentiated between ingredients from different Strophanthus species. Catillon won in 1888 pure substances from the Strophanthus species gratus, hispidus, niger and kombé. He regularly received crystalline products only from Strophanthus gratus, while the others, especially Strophanthus kombé, only supplied amorphous products. At the same time Arnaud was concerned with an arrow poison that the Somalis extracted from the wood of a tree called *Acokanthera ouabaio*. In 1888 he succeeded in isolating a crystalline active substance, which he called ouabain. Only a short time later, he found an identical active ingredient in an arrow poison made from Strophanthus gratus. The name g-Strophanthin for the Strophanthus gratus glycoside was introduced by Thoms in 1904 to distinguish it from the active ingredients of other Strophanthus species [Gilg 1904]. The glycoside found in the Strophanthus kombé investigated by Fraser was henceforth referred to as k-Strophanthin.

Ouabain, which is identical to g-Strophanthin, largely replaced k-Strophanthin preparations in the therapy of heart patients in France after the First World War as "Ouabain Arnaud". In Germany, clinical Strophanthus research only began at the beginning of the 20th century with a publication by Schedel. He refers to Fraser, because after his publication in 1885, *"a veritable flood of publications appeared on this new cardiac drug, a sign that the use of digitalis does not meet all requirements."* In his work published in 1904 Schedel reports on positive experiences with a Strophanthus gratus tincture containing g-Strophanthin (ouabain). He emphasizes the beneficial effects on respiratory distress (dyspnoea) and pulse in heart patients also observed by other clinicians [Schedel 1904].

~ ~ ~

When Fraser published his groundbreaking work on the effects of Strophanthus' active ingredients in 1885, drugs were usually produced in doctors' pharmacies and home pharmacies. But also herbalists, pedlars and quacks were allowed to sell products declared as remedies. There was practically no regulation and control of the production, quality and efficacy of drugs. The purity and efficacy of drugs depended on the skill and experience of the individual pharmacist. Most pharmacists were still familiar with the use of native medicinal plants such as Foxglove species. However, every pharmacist used recipes he had developed himself to manufacture his products. In order to ensure a minimum quality of medicines, official pharmacopoeias were already being compiled in many countries in the 18th century, listing drugs known to be effective and methods for their production and storage. The first German pharmacopoeia (DAB1) was published in 1872 and the Pharmacopoea Austriaca was valid in Austria from 1812. The United States Pharmacopeia has existed in America since 1820.

Dealing with tropical plants posed new challenges for pharmacists and doctors. There was no experience with the identification of plants and suitable plant parts (leaves, seeds) and methods of preparing suitable dosage forms. The chemical analysis was not yet at a level that would have enabled an exact determination of the active ingredient content of plants and extracts. Empirical testing was the rule, extreme quality differences of supposedly identical products the inevitable result.

The period at the end of the 19th century was a period of political and economic upheaval. Progress in many scientific disciplines has led to the *scientificisation* of therapeutic measures in medicine. Empiricism and tradition were replaced by science. Industrial companies based on research were founded. Companies such as Hoechst, Bayer, BASF, Sandoz, Ciba, E. R. Squibb and Sons (now Bristol-Myers Squibb) and Boehringer were all founded in the second half of the 19th century. They were all looking for attractive products. The production of medicines was a promising business field.

In 1851 Ernst Christian Friedrich Schering (1824-1889) founded a pharmacy in Berlin, which in 1864 became the *Chemische Fabrik Ernst Schering*, which boasted of offering *pure preparations*. The later gave rise to Schering AG, which today is part of the Bayer Group. The pharmacist Heinrich Emanuel Merck (1794 - 1855) had already started in 1827 selling isolated active ingredients from plants such as caffeine, cocaine, morphine and nicotine to other pharmacists, chemists and doctors. These activities were the cornerstone of the pharmaceutical and chemical company E. Merck Darmstadt. Merck's product range focused on active ingredients derived from tropical plants. Hoping for more valuable plants was the reason why botanists like John Kirk always participated in expeditions like the one from Livingstone to Mozambique. Their task was to look specifically for such plants.

The American Henry Wellcome (1853-1936) had a great personal interest in new developments in medicine, pharmacology and botany. He was convinced of the great potential of tropical plants for new drugs. In the 1870s he had been on the road in South America in search of plants containing quinine. In 1880, together with his partner Silas Burroughs, he founded the company Burroughs, Wellcome & Co in London. The young company was looking for new products. When Fraser reported on his therapeutic experiences with homemade

Strophanthus tinctures at the annual meeting of the British Medical Association in Cardiff in 1885, Henry Wellcome was also present. After an intensive discussion with Fraser, Wellcome decided to include the Strophanthus product in the product portfolio of his young company. Fraser supported Burroughs, Wellcome & Co with his knowledge of selecting suitable Strophanthus seeds and producing a tincture suitable for therapeutic use. Already in 1886 the new product *Tincture of Strophanthus* was on sale, which was sold at seven shillings per ounce in England and America. From 1887 the tincture was also marketed in Germany, Holland and other countries. The tincture was recommended in adults for the treatment of heart murmurs, nervous asthma, typhoid fever and pneumonia. With sweet syrup to mask the bitter taste it was also given to children.

Initially, it proved difficult to obtain sufficient quantities of suitable Strophanthus seeds for the industrial production of Strophanthus tinctures. Only the seeds of Strophanthus kombé were suitable for the production of the tincture developed by Fraser. However, seeds of unsuitable Strophanthus species were often delivered. With the help of John Buchanan, the British Consul of Malawi, Wellcome built a reliable supply chain [Hokkanen 2012]. In 1906, 16 tons of Strophanthus seeds worth 8,000 British pounds were exported from the British Protectorate in Central Africa to England. The seeds were harvested from wild plants. Cultivating the plants did not seem attractive enough. Other companies also began to market Strophanthus products. Some of these were of dubious quality. To distance himself from these, Wellcome advertised that its tincture corresponded to the original recipe of Fraser and was tested by him. Burroughs Wellcome made extensive use of medical and scientific literature in his advertising - especially Fraser's articles. From the beginning of 1886, reprints of Fraser's publications in *The Lancet* and *British Medical Journal* were used to promote the *Tincture of Strophanthus*. The authority of science is still used today by all pharmaceutical companies as an essential part of the marketing strategy for drugs. The *Tincture of Strophanthus* was a commercial success and founded the rapid growth of Burroughs, Wellcome & Co in the late 19th century.

Initially, no reliable information was available on suitable medical indications for the Strophanthus tincture. Fraser had described the diuretic effect, rapid onset of action and positive effects on edema and respiratory distress in a few patients. Fraser stressed in particular that *"strophanthin increases the action of the heart without raising blood pressure."* Further clinical and pharmacological investigations were necessary. As Burroughs Wellcome did not yet have its own laboratories, it made its tincture available to doctors and hospitals at home and abroad free of charge for experimental purposes. In 1894 the Wellcome Physiological Research Laboratories were founded, one of the first commercial research laboratories of their time.

In 1930 Burroughs Wellcome began selling digoxin preparations containing pure digoxin isolated from Digitalis lanata that very quickly became a great commercial success.

In America, E. R. Squibb and Sons was one of the first suppliers of Strophanthus products. Particularly popular was a chocolate-coated tablet of a mixture of Digitalis and Strophanthus extracts, which was sold at 16 cents per hundred pieces. The recommended dose for palpitations, smoking heart and as a heart tonic was one tablet every three to four hours. In Germany, Strophanthus preparations were developed by Boehringer Mannheim and E. Merck. In the absence of suitable research departments, these companies also made samples of pure Strophanthus extracts available to interested physicians and scientists for scientific investigations.

Info-Box Heart Glycosides

The drugs known as *heart-active glycosides* are also known as *cardiac glycosides* or *steroid glycosides*. *The* representatives of this class of chemical agents are found in numerous plant species. In addition to Foxglove species (Digitalis), these include Adonis rose (Adonis), Lily of the Valley (Convallaria majalis), Oleander (Nerium oleander) and the African lianas of the Strophanthus species and the African tree Acokanthera ouabaio. Approximately 200 active ingredients of this class are known. Of medical significance are the Digitalis derivatives digitoxin (from Digitalis purpurea), digoxin (from Digitalis lanata) and the Strophanthus derivatives k-Strophanthin (from Strophanthus kombé) and g-Strophanthin (from Strophanthus gratus), which is identical to the ouabain isolated from Acokanthera ouabaio. Chemically, the steroid glycosides are all constructed according to the same principle: a steroid framework similar to that of sexual hormones and bile acids is connected to a sugar chain consisting of one or more sugar residues. The steroid glycosides differ from each other by different sugar chains and different substituents on the steroid framework. The steroid skeleton is called *aglycon* or *genin*.

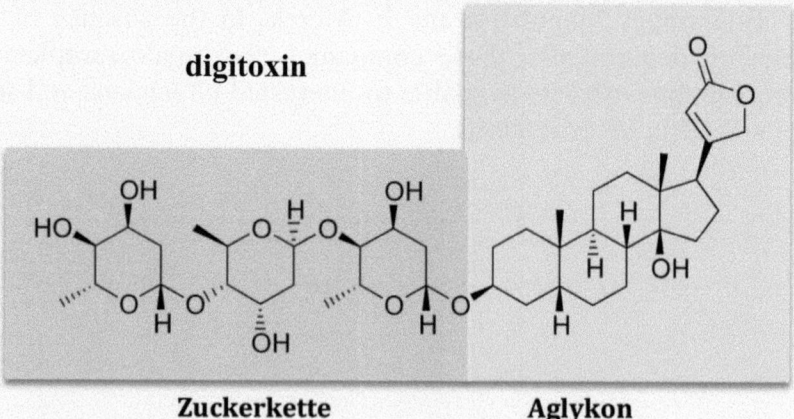

digitoxin

Zuckerkette   **Aglykon**

Digitoxose - Digitoxose - Digitoxose – Digitoxigenin

The Digitoxin contained in the Red Foxglove consists of the aglycon digitoxigenin and a sugar chain consisting of three units of digitoxose. The sugar chain of digoxin contained in Digitalis lanata also consists of three digitoxose units. It differs from digitoxin by a hydroxy group at the C-12 of the aglycon.

digoxin

Digitoxose - Digitoxose - Digitoxose - Digoxigenin

The structurally related steroid glycosides from the Strophanthus species - k-Strophanthin and g-Strophanthin - contain several hydroxyl groups in the aglycon. These cause a much higher water solubility than Digitalis derivatives. The g-Strophanthin found in Strophanthus gratus and Acokanthera ouabaio in English is named *Ouabain.*

k-Strophanthin

glucose - glucose - cymarose - k-strophanthidin

Today, this term is used exclusively in scientific literature. In contrast to the hydrolysis stable digoxin, digitoxin and ouabain, k-Strophanthin is very easily cleaved by acid and bases. The k-Strophanthin from Strophanthus kombé *(Kombetin)* used for therapeutic purposes therefore always contains small amounts of k-Strophanthin-β (produced by the elimination of one unit of glucose) and k-Strophanthin-α (produced by the elimination of two units of glucose). k-Strophanthin-α is identical to Cymarin obtained from the Adonis rose.

g-Strophanthin (Ouabain)

Rhamnose - g-Strophanthidin
(rhamnose - ouabagenin)

In addition to the natural active ingredients, semi-synthetic digoxin derivatives β -acetyl digoxin (trade name *Novodigal)* and β -methyl digoxin (trade name *Lanitop*) have also been successfully used in therapy. These derivatives have an improved absorption compared to digoxin. They release digoxin in the body and therefore have an effect identical to digoxin.

βacetyl digoxin

Pure chemical substances that are free of impurities tend to crystallize. If crystals a substance can be produced, this is a strong indication of the purity of the compound. If substances are present in amorphous, non-crystalline form, this is an indication of substance mixtures or contaminated substances. Crystalline k-Strophanthin has only been obtained in rare cases. The high susceptibility to hydrolysis means that parts of k-Strophanthin-β and Cymarin are always included. Therefore, unlike g-Strophanthin (ouabain), k-Strophanthin is always obtained as an amorphous product.

The exact chemical structure of cardiac glycosides was elucidated in the first decades of the 20th century. Decisive contributions came from Heinrich Kiliani (1855-1945), Nobel Prize winner Adolf Windaus (1875-1959), Rudolf Tschesche (1905-1981) and Arthur Stoll (1887-1971).

Schmiedeberg and the Digitaline

Withering was the founder of the systematic investigation of Digitalis effects. Building on Withering's work, generations of scientists have worked on Digitalis. Numerous new scientific findings did not change the indiscriminate use of Foxglove preparations in medical practice, nor did they change the frequency of poisoning. However, they laid the foundation for targeted investigations of the pharmacological properties of the active substances contained in Red Foxglove and related plants.

John Ferriar is ascribed the recognition that Digitalis primarily affects the heart. In 1799 he was the first to describe the pronounced effect of Digitalis extracts on heart function in his monograph on the Red Foxglove: *"Leaf extracts provide us with a means of regulating the heartbeat according to our wishes and to keep it at a given frequency as long as we judge it correctly."* In the same year, Thomas Beddoes published his observations that Digitalis increases the contractility of the heart muscle and only works in lung diseases if these are caused by heart failure.

There has been no lack of attempts to isolate the active substances contained in Digitalis plants. In 1835, the Société de Pharmacie de Paris awarded a prize of 500 francs for the best answer to the question:*"Are there in Digitalis purpurea one or more active ingredients to which the medicinal effects of this plant can be attributed?"* Because no one had isolated an active ingredient from the Red Foxglove, Société doubled the price five years later. In 1841 Homelle and Quevenne isolated a semi-crystalline product from Digitalis purpurea, which had biological effects, and received the Société award for it [Somberg 1985]. In 1864, the French chemist Nativelle isolated a crystalline substance, the *Digitaline Nativelle.* In 1875, Oswald Schmiedeberg in Strasbourg succeeded in obtaining a crystalline active substance from the leaves of the Red Foxglove, which he had collected in the Vosges.

He described this as *digitoxin*. As we know today, digitoxin is identical to Nativelle's digitaline. Schmiedeberg was one of the first scientists to investigate the effects of pure Digitalis active ingredients on animals. Schmiedeberg's work contributed significantly to the fact that in the second half of the 19th century it became clear that Digitalis active ingredients primarily affect the heart. This led to a sound understanding of the causes and progression of dropsy. A heart that is too weak at an advanced stage causes water retention in the lungs and other organs.

In the Franco-Prussian War of 1870/71, Alsace-Lorraine was annexed to the German Reich as *Reichsland Alsace-Lorraine*. In Strasbourg a German university was founded, which was to *"create an outpost of German culture and German spirit in an ancient German borderland, often damaged by romantic dilettantism and scientific superficiality"* [Bonah 2004]. Beyond national pathos, the aim was to build an elite university of natural sciences in the tradition of Enlightenment and committed to rational thinking. A special focus should be on basic medical sciences. Five of the eight chairs were in this area. These included two chairs of pharmacology and physiological chemistry, which were among the first of these disciplines in Germany. Highly qualified, experimentally working young scientists were appointed. Due to the successes of the close integration of interdisciplinary scientific research with medical education, the *Reich University of Strasbourg* (renamed *Kaiser Wilhelm University* in 1877) became the model for a general reorientation of German universities. Among others, Heinrich Wilhelm Waldeyer (1836-1921), the physiologist Friedrich Goltz (1834-1902), the pathologist Friedrich Daniel von Recklinghausen (1833-1910) and the pathologist Bernhard Naunyn (1839-1925) were appointed, all of whom contributed decisively to progress in medicine through their fundamental work. Felix Hoppe-Seyler was appointed to the Chair of Physiological Chemistry. Oswald Schmiedeberg, who held this position until he was expelled from France in 1918, was appointed Chair of Pharmacology.

Oswald Schmiedeberg (1838 - 1921) is regarded as the father of modern pharmacology. Born and raised in Latvia, he studied medicine at the University of Dorpat (Estonia) and completed his studies in 1866 with a doctoral thesis on the determination of chloroform in blood. Until 1869 he worked as assistant to his teacher Rudolf Buchheim, as his successor he took over the chair of pharmacology at the University of Dorpat in 1869. In 1872 he moved to Strasbourg.

Hoppe-Seyler and Schmiedeberg are among the most influential scientists in their disciplines. They have trained generations of scientists and thus made a decisive contribution to the establishment of rational pharmacology. In a 1883 publication, Schmiedeberg describes the relationship between physiological chemistry, pharmacology and medical clinic:

> "Physiological chemistry has to do with life under ordinary, therefore normal conditions, pathology with such life phenomena that occur under extraordinary or abnormal conditions of all kinds. Pharmacology conveys knowledge of the design and course of life processes under the influence of toxins. This classification, like all related branches of knowledge, is basically merely a division of labour. For the final result, it makes no difference whether pathology finally merges into pharmacology or vice versa and whether both merge with physiology to form a unified doctrine of life." [Bonah 2004].

Hoppe-Seyler and Schmiedeberg accelerated the foundation of their scientific disciplines by founding their own scientific journals. Hoppe-Seyler founded the *Zeitschrift für physiologische Chemie* (today: *Biological Chemistry*) in 1877. Together with Bernhard Naunyn and Edwin Klebs, Schmiedeberg initiated the *Archiv für experimentelle-Pathologie und Pharmakologie* (today: *Naunyn-Schmiedebergs Archives of Pharmacology)*. Both journals are still among the leading journals in their scientific disciplines.

Schmiedeberg's work is documented in more than 200 scientific publications. Active ingredients from Digitalis and related plants were a major focus of his research. In addition to digitoxin from the Red Foxglove (1874), he isolated other heart-active substances from Digitalis and related plant species such as lilies of the valley (Convallaria majalis) and oleanders (Nerium oleander). In addition, he also investigated the pharmacological effects of ingredients of African Strophanthus species, in particular that of Strophanthus kombé. Schmiedeberg and his team carried out detailed studies on the effect of cardiac glycosides on frog hearts with which they were able to experimentally prove the effect of these active substances on the heart. Together with Francis Williams and Heinrich Dreser, Schmiedeberg discovered the increase in the contraction force of the heart muscle by cardiac glycosides. Dreser later worked for Farbenfabriken Bayer in Leverkusen, where he played a key role in the development of Aspirin and Heroin.

Due to their similar basic chemical structure (all cardiac glycosides consist of a steroid framework to which sugar units are bound, see Info Box on cardiac glycosides) and their similar toxic effect on animal hearts, Schmiedeberg grouped all substances similar to Digitalis known to him into a group of pharmacological active substances, which he called *Digitaline-Group*. For Schmiedeberg, apart from quantitative differences, cardiac glycosides had such a *"similar effect on the heart that each of them appears to be a faithful copy of the other."* Albert Fraenkel spoke in 1933 of *"the great accomplishment of Schmiedeberg when he combined Strophanthin and all other glycosides with the same basic effect into the group of digitalis bodies. Despite all the differences of the individual Strophanthins among themselves and compared to the other Digitalis substances in the narrower... and further meaning ... it must be maintained that all substances belonging here are pharmacologically identical."* [Fraenkel 1933]. Schmiedeberg thus established the dogma still valid today that all cardio-active glycosides have qualitatively equal effects, which differ only quantitatively slightly from each other. As a result of this assessment, all cardiac glycosides, whether derived from Digitalis or Strophanthus, are still referred to as *Digitalis Glycosides in* scientific literature today.

In the second half of the 19th century, as in other countries, many industrial companies in Germany began producing and selling pharmaceuticals. This also included the sale of active ingredients derived from medicinal plants. Schmiedeberg developed close relationships with the pharmaceutical industry in Germany and starting in 1885 worked as a consultant for Boehringer Mannheim. At Schmiedeberg's suggestion, the company started working on cardiac glycosides. In 1889 Boehringer launched an active ingredient derived from the African Strophanthus species Strophanthus kombé as *Strophanthin Boehringer*. Schmiedeberg provided Boehringer with several active ingredients, including Strophanthin. The water solubility of Strophanthin made it possible to use aqueous solutions of the active ingredient for pharmacological investigations of frog and mammalian hearts, a decisive advantage over the water-insoluble active ingredients of Foxglove. The rapid onset of the effect after Strophanthin application was an additional advantage. Thus, Strophanthin became the standard preparation for the study of the effects of Digitalis glycosides, a function which it still performs today in current science.

The quality of Digitalis preparations

At the beginning of the 20th century, the most important cardiac glycosides - digitoxin, digoxin, k-Strophanthin, g-Strophanthin (ouabain) - were known as pure substances. Pharmacological studies had shown the effects on the heart. In clinical practice, however, Digitalis and Strophanthus preparations remained controversial. As in Withering's time, the therapeutic effects were not reliable and hardly reproducible. Symptoms of poisoning and even deaths were still very frequent. Clinicians had not yet reached agreement on diseases in which cardiac glycosides are appropriate. The products have continued to be used in a wide range of diseases.

Ackerknecht sees the attempt to regard new drugs as a panacea as a general habit of doctors: *"Doctors have always been under terrible pressure, and despite all the progress made, they are still forced to do something about diseases, while the actual means of combating them are limited. When an effective drug appears, it is soon used far beyond its intended purpose, driven by hope and despair. According to Corvisart's[2] old adage that new drugs always produce positive results, and because of people's infamous "autistic" habits, it takes decades to discover the actual situation. This seems to be the root of the desire for panaceas"* [Ackerknecht 1962]. In the case of Digitalis active ingredients, it took more than 100 years to *discover the actual situation* and to clarify the use of these active ingredients. As in Withering's time, one of the main problems was the quality of the preparations used.

---

[2] Jean-Nicolas Corvisart (1755 - 1821), French cardiologist and personal physician of Napoleon.

Albert Fraenkel (1864-1938), a phyysician working in Badenweiler and conducting research in Heidelberg at the time, described the situation of cardiac glycosides at the beginning of the 20th century:

"It is a fact known to us physicians and much lamented by us that the effectiveness of galenic Digitalis preparations varies according to their provenance, and we know that this difference is due to the drug's varying content of active ingredients. The year and location of the plant, the age and preparation of the leaves and the time at which they are collected are the factors on which the content of an infusion or tincture of active substance depends. It is not without good reason that individual pharmacies in almost every region and city are called upon to supply particularly good preparations. ... The same applies to the official Strophanthus preparations. For the various Strophanthus drugs of overseas origin, the content of active ingredients varies considerably more than is the case with the domestic, better characterized Digitalis purpurea. Their therapeutic value is assessed very differently by the various authors and, what must be particularly noted, in the different countries. One is probably not sufficiently clear about the fact that the unequal evaluation of the means might depend also here to the largest part on fluctuations of the preparations in the content of active substance" [Fraenkel 1902].

"For internal Digitalis therapy, in addition to the galenic preparations, the powder and infus, to which are added the drinks and dialysates, we have the pure bodies at our disposal. The use of the pure bodies per os has been tried many times in Germany, but mostly abandoned. In France, Digitalia Nativelle, an impure preparation containing Schmiedebergs Digitoxin as its main ingredient, is widely used. ... A faster and more energetic effect than with good galenic preparations cannot be achieved with Digitoxin and other pure bodies." [Fraenkel 1907].

Albert Fraenkel, born in 1864 in Mußbach an der Weinstraße, studied medicine in Munich and Strasbourg and graduated in 1888. After working as an assistant physician in Munich, Fraenkel settled in Badenweiler in 1891 as a spa physician. He founded the sanatorium *Villa Hedwig* for the treatment of internal diseases and in 1903 the sanatorium *Villa Paul* for lung patients. In addition to his work in Badenweiler, Fraenkel worked at the Institute of Pharmacology at the Ruprecht-Karls University in Heidelberg from the winter semester of 1893/94 and was involved in the pharmacology of cardiac glycosides. In 1920 he moved to Heidelberg. There he worked as a physician at the hospital for tuberculosis patients in Rohrbach. In 1927 he founded the internistic *Mittelstands-Sanatorium Speyererhof* and from then on he was active as its medical director. In recognition of his achievements, Fraenkel was appointed full honorary professor of the University of Heidelberg in 1928 with a teaching position for tuberculosis. After the seizure of power in 1933, the National Socialists dismissed the Jew Fraenkel from all offices. In September 1938, his licensure was also revoked. Three months later he died in Heidelberg at the age of 74.

During his studies at the Kaiser-Wilhelms-Universität in Strassburg, Albert Fraenkel learned the principles of medicine based on scientific knowledge. From Oswald Schmiedeberg, he not only learnt the importance of pharmacology for rational medicinal research. From Schmiedeberg he also took over his scientific field of work, the treatment of heart diseases with cardiac glycosides. For Fraenkel, the neglect of dosage and with it the numerical registration of the effect was a *curse on the application of Digitalis.* He considered the demand for a standardized dosage to be a *mental defect in the field of pharmacological therapy* [Fraenkel 1936]. He found the request of some pharmacologists grotesque to standardise the dose of a drug in grams per kilogram body weight. According to Fraenkel, the dose of a cardiac glycoside should always be adjusted to the patient's needs. Digitalis preparations with known and constant potency were an indispensable prerequisite for this. One of his first publications dealt with *the physiological dosage of Digitalis preparations* [Fraenkel 1902].

Fraenkel described the necessity of experimentally determining and standardizing the potency of Digitalis preparations. The chemical analysis was not yet able to do this. Although the active substances could be obtained in pure form and could be characterized by different color reactions with sulfuric acid, a quantitative determination in plants and extracts was not yet technically possible. Clear therapeutic results with Strophanthus tincture could only be achieved if uniform tinctures of standardized potency were used.

Fraenkel therefore opted for a pharmacological test to determine the efficacy of Digitalis preparations. In order to experimentally determine the potency of a substance , there must be an effect specific to the substance, which dose-dependent always shows the same effect in a reproducible manner. For the Digitalis extracts, Fraenkel chose the systolic standstill of the frog heart, a test which he had learned from Schmiedeberg in Strasbourg and which, in his opinion, *"does everything that can only be demanded of a pharmacological test object"*.

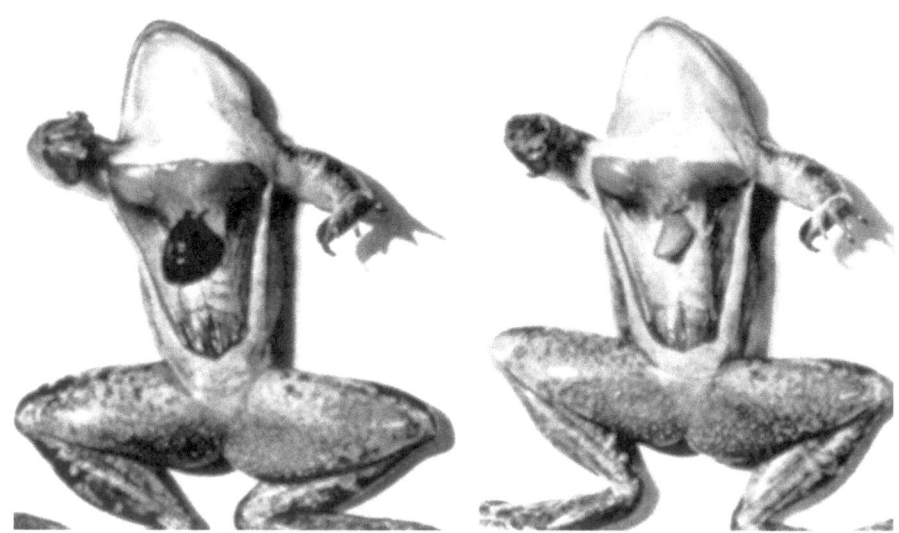

Frog heart in diastole   **Frog heart in systole**
In the diastole the heart is filled with blood, in the systole it is emptied

Fraenkel defined *"frog-unit" as the amount of a Digitalis body that is sufficient for a frog weighing about 30 g to bring the heart to a systolic standstill within half an hour.* Equal amounts of fluid were always injected into the lymphatic sacs. The frogs were weighed, the increasing dosage given in absolute quantities and converted into 100 g frog. The minimum dose, which led to systolic cardiac arrest within half an hour, was also given per 100 g of frog.

With this system it was possible to carry out comparative studies of different preparations and to indicate their effect in frog-units, which allowed a numerical comparison of the potency levels. Fraenkel determined the effectiveness of different preparations and came to frightening results. The potencies of various Digitalis tinctures showed differences of up to 400 percent. Even more dramatic were the differences in Strophanthus preparations. Fraenkel found differences of up to 6,000 percent. These measurement results prove that the cardiac glycoside preparations used at the beginning of the 20th century often contained ineffective concentrations of active substance, which explains the very different treatment successes reported by many physicians.

Fraenkel reports that *"doctors abroad, especially in France, England and Holland, make more extensive use of Strophanthus preparations"* than in Germany. He also tested preparations from there and concluded that *"the tablets from Burroughs, Wellcome & Co. which are widely used in England and America and which are only gradually becoming established in Germany as a result of the resistance of pharmacists are particularly effective"*.

The industrially produced *Digitoxin Merck* also proved to be particularly effective. Fraenkel therefore pleaded for the production of these drugs in *large chemical companies.* The industry should offer galenic products with a certain titer using an appropriate method or, similar to vaccines, the state should also set up test centres for Digitalis preparations. It is not surprising that this proposal met with strong opposition from pharmacists.

Albert Fraenkel was not the first researcher to investigate the problem of purity and potency of cardiac glycosides. This problem was worked on worldwide at the beginning of the 20th century. Alexander Berghaus and Rolf Winau have described in detail the development of the standardization of Digitalis preparations and the problems to be solved [Berghaus 1982]. The frog method has been optimized many times. Test systems on other animal species were added. The experiments culminated in the realization that internationally comparable statements on the potency of certain Digitalis preparations could only be achieved with methodologically completely unified measuring methods, and that a uniform measure of effectiveness had to be found.

In 1922, the President of the Hygiene Organization of the League of Nations initiated an investigation into which remedies, apart from the sera and bacterial products, required an internationally recognized biological assessment. Digitalis and Strophanthus preparations were among these remedies. A conference convened in Edinburgh in 1923 was intended to create stable preparations on the one hand and reliable biological research methods on the other. At this conference, three calibrated Digitalis powders were selected, which served for two years as reference substances for a wide variety of valuation methods. The results were discussed at a second conference in Geneva in 1925 and two agreements were reached:

- An internationally recognized Digitalis powder, mixed from ten different powders, should be produced, which should be adjusted with the help of a test on cats and made available to all interested parties.

- The cat method and the frog method are permitted as methods for determining the potency.

No uniform test method was agreed. Instead, the Geneva Conference proposed that Digitalis preparations should not deviate in their potency by more than 25% from the standard preparation.

At first, these efforts did little to change the variety of qualitatively very different products on the market. In 1936 Fraenkel was frustrated to find that *"the variety of so-called substitutes flooding markets and doctors around the world is in inverse proportion to the level of rational Digitalis therapy. It's gone down and there's a lot of confusion. Overdosing there, underdosing here. The colliery will be paid by the insufficient."* To protect against the enormous fluctuations in the active ingredient content of the preparations, Fraenkel suggested using pure active ingredients with a constant potency instead of tinctures. He was well aware that these highly effective substances can quickly lead to dramatic side effects if not dosed carefully. *"It is understandable that the practice is reluctant to approach these very effective, but all the more dangerous substances with careless dosage and initially still adheres to the galenic preparations, about which thousands of experiences are available."*

In 1906, pure active ingredients were offered in Germany by Boehringer Mannheim *(Strophanthin Boehringer;* active ingredient k-Strophanthin), by E. Merck *(Digitoxin Merck*; active ingredient digitoxin and *Strophanthin crystallisatum nach Thoms;* active ingredient ouabain) and Kali-Chemie *(Purostrophan*; active ingredient ouabain). For his further research, Fraenkel chose the *Strophanthin Boehringer*, with which he was familiar from his time in Strasbourg and which was made available to scientists free of charge by Boehringer Mannheim. It was well soluble in water, showed a fast-acting and long-lasting effect and was therefore better suited for experiments than digitoxin. This is not water soluble and has a slow onset of effect.

Intravenous Strophanthin therapy

At the beginning of the 20th century, pharmacology, still young and influenced by Schmiedeberg, concentrated on the investigation of the toxic effects of substances on healthy animals. The frog method for determining the active value of Digitalis preparations also measured the toxicity of the active ingredients. Fraenkel put the resulting limitations in principle into question

> *"Are we at all entitled to conclude from the toxic effect of a Digitalis body on the frog's heart on its therapeutic effect on humans?"*

This central question as to whether the healing and toxic effects are causally related and even follow the same dose-response relationships, i.e. whether a remedy is always also poison, has occupied future generations of scientists intensively and for cardiac glycosideshas not yet been conclusively answered even today. When using drugs for the therapy of diseases, it is necessary to choose the dosage in such a way that the therapeutic effects appear, but toxic effects are excluded. Toxic effects are not suitable for the study of therapeutic effects. Effects and parameters must be chosen which are characteristic for the therapeutic effect of the substances.

In animal experiments, low doses of cardiac glycosides led to an increase in blood pressure and a slowdown in heart rate. In his study "Über die Digitaliswirkung am gesunden Menschen" (On the effects of Digitalis on healthy people) Fraenkel therefore investigated the effect of Strophantus tinctures on the blood pressure and pulse of healthy people [Fraenkel 1908]. The surprising result was that blood pressure did not rise after application of Strophanthin, unlike in animal experiments. Contrary to the principles of his teacher Schmiedeberg, Fraenkel from his studies derived the demand to study cardiac glycosides preferentially on sick patients: *"If Withering had used ex-*

perimental pharmacological methods, the healing power of the Digitalis would have escaped him."

for Albert Fraenkel availability of pure preparations with known and constant potency was a necessary but by no means sufficient condition for a reliable effect of cardiac glycosides in human therapy. It was equally important to work out an exact dosage of the preparations for the patients and to determine how much of the active substance administered reaches the site of its effect in the human body. In today's nomenclature it was therefore necessary to examine the dose, absorption, distribution and excretion of the active substance. Fraenkel saw no way to investigate these problems with orally administered preparations. For *"the path from the stomach to the heart is long, the loss of effective substance and thus also the duration of the effect is unpredictable."* [Fraenkel 1933]. There was only one way to avoid the insurmountable difficulties of oral administration based on the examination methods known at the time: intravenous injection. This was known and customary from pharmacological investigations on animals. The test substances were also administered by injection when determining the frog-value. At the beginning of the 20th century, however, only a few doctors had ever tried to administer active substances intravenously to people. There were general reservations. Schmiedeberg also doubted the usefulness of the method and considered it too dangerous. He feared the increase in blood pressure known from animal experiments. As Fraenkel became aware of Kottmann's attempts to administer *Digalen* - a water-insoluble glycerine extract of Digitalis offered by Hoffmann-LaRoche - intravenously to patients [Kottmann 1905] he decided to dare the experiment. He was convinced that Boehringer's k-Strophanthin was a preparation that was much better suited for intravenous application than *Digalen*. *"It was precisely this combination with sustained effectiveness that made Strophanthin particularly suitable for intravenous therapy. The animal experiments were mainly carried out with Strophanthin Boehringer. We therefore decided to use this preparation, which we knew is very effectively and evenly, for human use."*

The head of the University Hospital in Strasbourg, Ludolf von Krehl, allowed Fraenkel - contrary to Schmiedeberg's explicit warning that Strophanthin lacked the *"toxic effects on the animal heart"* compared to digitoxin - to investigate the intravenous application of *Strophanthin Boehringer* (k-Strophanthin) in patients. In the winter of 1905, Fraenkel and Georges Schwartz, assistant physician at the clinic, examined the effects of intravenous Strophanthin therapy on 25 heart patients. At the 23rd Congress for Internal Medicine in Munich from April 23 to 26, 1906, he reported on the groundbreaking successes achieved:

> "Even the first attempts with the right doses showed the brilliant success of the new method: the speed and strength of the effect. From the internal therapy we are accustomed to the gradual onset of the Digitalis effect, which we can never predict exactly according to time and intensity; here we are faced with an effect that starts within 3 - 4 minutes and which we master. Under our eyes the switching of the pathological cycle to the norm takes place. The patient's pulse becomes fuller, his breathing slower and a flood of urine breaks out in such a short time that we have never been able to reach it. A patient who before the procedure was apathetically suffering from the effects of CO_2 overload recovered quickly, the other, who presented the symptoms of severe cardiac dyspnea and the anxiety and restlessness caused by it, calmed down and many after a single injection already found the sleep they had had to deprive themselves of for weeks. If every happily performed Digitalis treatment appears to be a triumph of medical art, this rapid help through intravenous injection of the drug acts like a miracle cure and the physician is faced with an equally important pharmacological and clinical experiment [Fraenkel 1906].

This grandiose success had its price. The tests had not gone off without problems. There have been deaths. In one of his last letters to Schwartz on November 15, 1938, Fraenkel wrote: *"Dear Georg, do you actually still remember the restaurant in which we before*

Christmas 1905 drowned the terror of the first Strophanthin death and you encouraged me so well?" The reference to the *first* death indicates further deaths. 1907 Fraenkel reports in a study *about intravenous Strophanthin injections in cardiac patients* about another death as a consequence of too high a dosage. The patient had received 3 mg Strophanthin within 29 hours [Fraenkel 1907].

In the following years Fraenkel systematically investigated the indications for which intravenous Strophanthin is indicated. Fraenkel saw his special significance especially in conditions of acute heart failure. Here, intravenous application often saved lives. In 1908 Vaquez introduced intravenous Strophanthin therapy in France using *Ouabain Arnaud*, which contained ouabain, and received fierce criticism. Until then, *Digitaline Nativelle* was used as the standard cardiac glycoside in France. Vaquez was accused of wanting to *dethrone* the digitoxin, which led Vaquez to a vigorous replica [Vaquez 1917]. Vaquez determined clear differences in effect between ouabain and Digitalis preparations. Ouabain had a stronger effect on the contractility of the heart muscle, while the Digitalis preparations had a stronger influence on transition and excitability. Vaquez further differentiated between a diastolic Digitalis and a systolic ouabain effect. He also distinguished between right- and left-failure. For right-ventricle failure he used Digitalis preparations, for left-ventricle failure he used ouabain. According to Fraenkel, there was no sufficient experimental foundation for such differentiations.

With reference to numerous pharmacological investigations - which, as was customary in pharmacology at the time, had all been carried out at relatively high doses - and to his own clinical observations with Boehringer's k-Strophanthin, Fraenkel rejected Vaquez' differentiations. There would be no qualitative differences in effect between the Digitalis and Strophanthus cardiac glycosides; *"only quantitative, no qualitative differences are possible"*. He insisted that there is not a single *"specific therapeutic Digitalis or Strophanthin effect"* [Fraenkel 1933].

Fraenkel refused oral administration of Strophanthin preparations because of the known sensitivity of the k-Strophanthin, which leads to the decomposition of the active ingredient in the stomach. He excluded the official Strophanthus tincture from his criticism: *"In order to avoid misunderstandings, it should be expressly pointed out that all this applies only to Strophanthin, but not to Strophanthus tincture. The alcoholic extract that FRASER has already produced is superior to Strophanthin on an enteral route, but cannot compete intravenously with it."* [Fraenkel 1936]. He saw the large number of contradictory reports on the effects of orally administered Strophanthus preparations as confirmation of his experience that *"there is only one safe entry port for Strophanthin"* - intravenous injection.

But it took more than three decades until intravenous Strophanthin therapy was generally accepted and used. Based on the correspondence between Albert Fraenkel and Boehringer Mannheim, which is accessible in the Mannheim City Archive, Egon Dietz has described in detail the long and difficult process of implementing intravenous Strophanthin therapy and the development of the product *Kombetin* marketed by Boehringer [Dietz 2004].

Kombetin

After Fraser's publications on the effects of Strophanthus kombé extracts Boehringer Mannheim was one of the first companies in Germany to study this new active substance. At the suggestion of Oswald Schmiedeberg efforts were made to produce a pure preparation of the Strophanthus kombé active ingredient by folowing Fraser's specifications. Similar to Burroughs Wellcome, it was difficult for Boehringer to obtain suitable Strophanthus seeds. Of the more than 40 known species, five different species had been found in German East Africa alone. Boehringer succeeded in installing a methodology that made it possible to distinguish Strophanthus kombé seeds from those of other species. The active ingredient contained in Strophanthus kombé dissolved in sulfuric acid produces a characteristic green solution. This sulphuric acid sample made it possible to distinguish the kombé seeds from those of other species. For practical purposes, 100 seeds were randomly collected from a delivery of seeds to be tested and subjected to a sulphuric acid sample. After isolation of the Strophanthin, the product was subjected to another test. Hydrolysis was used to determine the aglycone of k-Strophanthin, k-Strophanthidin. Only if at least 90 percent of the theoretically calculated amount of k-Strophanthidin was contained was the tested delivery accepted as a suitable starting material for the production of *Strophanthin Boehringer*. From 1889 Boehringer marketed the product to pharmacies and made it available to scientists free of charge for experimental purposes. Albert Fraenkel was also among the recipients. He met with the company's Executive Board in Mannheim on March 14, 1906. He reported on his clinical trials with *Strophanthin Boehringer*. He intended to present the results at the Internist Congress in Munich in April. Fraenkel was convinced that his report would be very well received and that many doctors soon would adopt the intravenous Strophanthin therapy. It was therefore necessary for Boehringer to provide ready-to-use ampoules for intravenous injection.

Boehringer Mannheim had no experience in the production of sterile injection solutions, but agreed to produce samples. Fraenkel's proposal to present the product at the Internist Congress in Munich was not accepted. There were doubts in Mannheim that the effort involved would be worthwhile. In addition, fundamental production problems had to be clarified, which was hardly possible in the few weeks leading up to the congress. The injection solution filled in glass ampoules had to be sterile and stable in storage. The only known method of sterilisation at that time was the heating of the ampoule contents, a not unproblematic process due to the known susceptibility of k-Strophanthin to hydrolysis. To minimise the hydrolysis of active ingredient, Boehringer therefore used a special glass that only emitted a small amount of alkali. The sterilization process and storage stability were optimized in test series. The potency of the solutions was determined by Fraenkel using the frog method. It turned out that one-minute heating made the injection solution germ-free without affecting the potency. Boehringer ordered the first product batches from the Berlin company Kade. At the beginning of 1907 the product was offered under the brand name *Kombetin* for 2.50 Marks per 12 ampoules with an active ingredient content of 1 mg each in 1 cc solution. It could be obtained from the company Kade and directly from Boehringer. Contrary to Fraenkel's expectations, however, his Munich lecture did not lead to any noteworthy demand. The resistance to Kombetin and intravenous Strophanthin therapy was manifold. Quality problems, deaths and ignorance of the correct injection technique impaired rapid acceptance of intravenous Strophanthin therapy.

Only a few months after its market launch, Boehringer became aware of *"without exception unpleasant side effects"* when using Kombetin. Checks revealed that ampoules contaminated had been delivered by Kade. Boehringer then invested in the in-house production of the ampoules. For quality control purposes, samples from each batch were tested by Fraenkel for their potency.

Thoms in 1904 had described the production and properties of a pure, crystalline active ingredient from Strophanthus gratus. This had already been identified by Arnaud in 1888 and was identical to the ouabain found in Acokanthera ouabaio. For differentiation from the amorphous active substance obtained by Fraser from Strophanthus kombé, Thoms named the Strophanthus gratus active substance as *"g-Strophanthin"* and the amorphous product from Strophanthus kombé as *"k-Strophanthin"*. E. Merck marketed the g-Strophanthin under the name *Strophanthin crystallisatum nach Thoms.* - From 1914 onwards, Merck routinely had its Digitalis and Strophanthus preparations tested at the Pharmacological Institute of the University of Erlangen using a modified frog test [E. Merck 1914]. - The majority of pharmacologists preferred the crystalline g-Strophanthin because the amorphous k-Strophanthin had the reputation of being contaminated. Criticism of amorphous Strophanthin also came from France. There, the crystalline *"Ouabain Arnaud"* was preferred and a lower quality of amorphous products was criticized. At the time, Fraenkel himself did not yet know from which Strophanthus species Boehringer produced the *Strophanthin Boehringer.* In response to his request for information about the *origin and nature* of *Strophanthin Boehringer,* Mannheim reacted evasively and merely informed him in February 1907, referring to trade secrets, that it was an amorphous Strophanthin which was not obtained from Strophanthus gratus.

There were also official reservations against the amorphous Strophanthin. In May 1908 Fraenkel wrote to Boehringer: *"It has come to my attention that in the Pharmacopoeia Commission a trend has asserted itself against the amorphous Strophanthin and that apparently a tendency exists to only list cryst. Strophanthin in the pharmacopoeia. Prof. Thoms himself is a member of the Reich Health Council."* It is therefore not surprising that after the outbreak of the First World War medical personnel in the German army by order of the ambulance corps exclusively used ouabain solutions to treat heart failure and not Kombetin. After the war, ouabain from army stocks dominated the market for several years. Chemische Fabrik Güstrow, part of Kali-Chemie, had launched its own ouabain preparation under the name *Purostrophan.* This was advertised with the argument that it is the purer product. It was falsely claimed that the g-Strophanthin Thoms and the k-Strophanthin Boehringer were two *"chemically identical bodies of merely different physical properties"* and that, unlike Boehringer, the purer, crystalline form was used.

However, the biggest commercial competition for Kombetin was not the products of other companies. It was the pharmacies. They purchased Strophanthin in substance from Boehringer or other companies such as Merck and Schuchard and produced their own injection solutions. Safe sterilization while maintaining the efficacy of these proprietary products was not always possible, an uncertainty factor that put an additional strain on the reputation of Strophanthin. The constantly increasing volume of home-made injection solutions in pharmacies finally prompted Boehringer to stop the sale of pure Strophanthin in 1933.

There was criticism of Kombetin not only from the commercial side, but also from the scientific community. There were warnings of intravenous therapy, there were negative publications, there were deaths. In December 1908 Boehringer quoted in a letter to Fraenkel from a publication summarising the criticism:

"Even the Strophanthus seeds, which were only used a few decades ago, have not been able to escape modern efforts to improve. Here, too, a substance has been found that is both chemically pure and practically applicable: Strophanthin. However, it seems to be a rather dangerous drug. Although the shaking frosts that were initially observed during its application have now been avoided by sterile preparation of the solution, so many unpleasant incidents and even deaths have become known in the short time since we used the product that we must strongly advise the greatest caution in its application. Moreover, this drug can only be administered intravenously, which means that the path to general practice is probably completely closed."

Severe side effects and deaths were a major problem at the beginning of intravenous Strophanthin therapy. The cause was too high doses, partly caused by too fast injections and too short intervals for multiple injections. *Strophanthin cardiac death* was a phenomenon feared by doctors. Historically, as in Withering's time, Digitalis preparations were administered in very high doses, which according to current knowledge were close to or even above the limit of toxic doses. Fraenkel had also worked at the Strasbourg clinic with a high dose of 1 mg, but soon reduced it to 0.75 mg. However, high doses were often maintained in the early years of intravenous Strophanthin therapy. Therefore, the official *safety limit* for Strophanthin in the German Pharmacopoeia was finally set at five milligrams per day. This daily dose is still 500 - 1,000 percent higher than the daily dose of 0.5 to 1 mg that was later considered reasonable. Based on his practical experience with Kombetin, Fraenkel also reduced his recommended dose to 0.5 mg. In 1914, he recommended Boehringer to reduce the size of the ampoules to 0.5 ccm accordingly. For marketing reasons, the company refused. It was not until 1925 that the wish of many physicians was accepted and a 0.5 ccm ampoule was offered in addition to the 1 ccm ampoule. Years later, ampoules with 0.25 ccm were added. In later decades, Boehringer added dextrose-diluted injection solutions to its product range, which, due to their larger volume, helped prevent poisoning caused by too rapid injections. The fear of the nightmare *Strophanthin cardiac death* remained a constant companion of Stropanthin until the end of intravenous therapy.

However, the main obstacle to the introduction of intravenous Strophanthin therapy were persistent general reservations about intravenous injection and doctors' ignorance of the correct injection technique. The use of the syringe was particularly difficult for doctors in private practice. The technique of intravenous injection was not part of medical training. Very often the vein was not hit and injected intramuscularly. This led to severe pain and the fear of the doctor and patient of this technique was correspondingly high. There was talk of *vein horror*. Fraenkel formulated the first *Instructions for the technical execution of injections*, which were added to the Kombetin ampoules from 1908. The manual was revised in 1917. It was included in all Strophanthin packs until 1959.

Fraenkel made a decisive contribution to the acceptance of intravenous Strophanthin therapy in 1927 with the foundation of the internal sanatorium *Mittelstand-Sanatoriums Speyererhof.* The desire for a clinical home for intravenous Strophanthin therapy was the central motive for the construction of the Speyererhof. Located below the Königstuhl in Heidelberg, this sanatorium, built with financial support from Boehringer Mannheim, soon became the training centre for generations of doctors in the application of intravenous Strophanthin therapy. The cardiac patients were not only treated at Speyererhof with intravenous Strophanthin therapy but also prepared for a life with chronic heart failure. Fraenkel wrote some *life rules for cardiac patients after successful treatment of cardiac insufficiency* and thus integrated intravenous Strophanthin therapy into a comprehensive overall therapeutic concept.

From 1930, Fraenkel regularly held several-day courses at the Speyererhof, during which he taught the scientific principles of intravenous Strophanthin therapy and the technique of intravenous injection. Albert Fraenkel successfully completed his efforts for intravenous Strophanthin therapy with a comprehensive monograph on Strophanthin, which had been planned for a long time and was finally completed in 1933. In a 1934 review of *"Strophanthin Therapy"* published in the Deutsches Archiv für klinische Medizin, it says:

> "The best connoisseur of Strophanthin therapy has crowned his life's work with this book. For the immense own experience, paired with the knowledge and critical use of the entire literature, has enabled the author to fulfil his task in a perfect manner. The whole essay is conducted in the spirit of Naunyn's word, which the author has placed at the top of his explanations: Healing will be science or it will not be at all."

The advanced training courses at Spyererhof, Fraenkels Strophanthin monograph and the cessation of the marketing of the Strophanthin

substance to pharmacies led to the economic success of the Kombetin, which Boehringer had long hoped for, starting around 1935. The
extension of indications to ischemic heart diseases (angina pectoris,
coronary heart disease) and myocardial infarction by Ernst Edens
have contributed significantly to this success. After years of stagnati-
on at a frustratingly low level, sales of Kombetin multiplied. In the
first three decades after its market launch, Boehringer Mannheim sold
only a few thousand packages of Kombetin per year, which did not
cover the associated costs. In March 1907 Boehringer wrote to Fraenkel, *"For us, the profit on Strophanthin remains; this in turn is very
limited by the fact that the single dose is a very minimal one, so that
10,000 injections have to be made before 10 g of Strophanthin are
consumed, which we sell for 10 Marks."* One year later it reports: *"In
this year, the proceeds were far from covering our costs for separate
prints, samples of doctors, etc.".* In 1926, *"29.4 % of sales were spent
on advertising Strophanthin, although on average only 15 % were
used for other preparations."* In May 1932 Boehringer was pleased to
announce to Fraenkel *"that sales in Strophanthin ampoules have risen
quite satisfactorily in recent months".* According to Boehringer's internal calculations, approximately 100,000 patients were treated with
Kombetin in 1932. No data on sales or patient numbers of competing
ouabain ampoules *(Strophanthin crystallisatum nach Thoms* from
Merck, *Purostrophan* from Chemische Fabrik Güstrow and Kali
Chemie) are available.

Kombetin's success was limited to Germany. Boehringer's efforts to
market the product in other countries failed. The company's New
York office, Rare Chemicals, applied to the Council on Pharmacy and
Chemistry of the American Medical Association for the official introduction of Strophanthin-Boehringer in 1936. The application was
rejected - probably for political reasons. Students of Fraenkel, who as
Jews had had to leave Nazi Germany, reported on *"doctrinarism and
prejudice against any progress coming from Germany."* This is not
surprising, given the fact that medicine, as the *New German Medicine*
in the Third Reich, had subjected itself to the Nazi ideology of social
Darwinian eugenics. In addition to politically motivated rejection,

there was also a fundamental rejection of intravenous therapy in the USA, of which Groedel reported in a letter to Fraenkel in 1935. *"The preconceived opinion is an almost insurmountable resistance here."* Fraenkel undertook numerous Boehringer-funded lecture tours, especially to England, Switzerland and Italy to promote intravenous Strophanthin therapy and Kombetin. But even in these countries it was not possible to overcome the aversion to intravenous administration of the drug. Intravenous Strophanthin therapy remained a primarily German phenomenon.

Albert Fraenkel was firmly integrated into the marketing strategy for Kombetin. Immediately after the Internistenkongress 1906 in Munich, reprints of the Fraenkel lecture were printed for advertising purposes. The same procedure was followed for later publications. In his work, Fraenkel always referred to the Kombetin and distanced himself from ouabain-based products. During the First World War, Fraenkel worked as a medical officer in the German Army. His patients included high-ranking military personnel in which he used Kombetin to break the monopoly of g-Strophanthin Thoms. In 1914 Fraenkel wrote an advertising text which was used by Boehringer in a letter to doctors in German, Swiss and Austrian health resorts. Fraenkel's scientific authority was also used in the technical instructions for carrying out injections included in the Kombetin packs, which bore his name.

Albert Fraenkel has been compensated by Boehringer Mannheim for his various activities for Kombetin. In the early years of the cooperation, the company reimbursed Fraenkel for the testing of the ampoules produced. For the year 1909, 140 Marks were paid for 14 tests. From 1923 Fraenkel received a share in the turnover of 10 Pfennig per 100 ampoules. This was raised to 25 Pfennig per 100 ampoules in 1925 and doubled to 50 Pfennig in 1929. In 1933, the Nazis banned Fraenkel from all offices. Thus, the share in Kombetin sales was Fraenkel's only remaining income. Boehringer increased its share of sales to 60 Pfennig per 100 ampoules and also assured his wife of a share of sales in the event of her husband's death. From then on, invoicing was no longer done annually but monthly.

Intravenous Strophanthin therapy initiated by Albert Fraenkel was practiced in Germany until the end of the 1990s.

Ernst Edens - The Treatment of Angina Pectoris

In addition to Albert Fraenkel, the Dusseldorf clinician Ernst Edens in particular has studied intensively the scobe and limitations of intravenous Strophanthin therapy. Ernst Edens, born 1876 in Rendsburg, studied medicine in Kiel, Berlin and Munich. In 1910 he habilitated in Munich as assistant to the internist Friedrich von Müller. In 1916 he took over the management of the Luisenheim Sanatorium in St. Blasien in the Black Forest. From 1925 to 1931 he was head of the Ebenhausen Sanatorium near Munich. In 1931 Edens was appointed Full Professor of Internal Medicine and Director of the Medical Clinic in Dusseldorf, where he worked until his death on March 19, 1944.

In his clinical work, Edens had observed that the effects on patients were also very different when using Digitalis preparations with constant potency. From this experience he already in 1920 had derived the rule *"Every heart has its own Digitalis dose"*. The effect on animal's heart could not easily be transferred to humans. Animal experiments have led to valuable insights into the absorption, distribution and excretion of the active substances. But just like Fraenkel, Eden was aware of the fundamental limitations of pharmacological investigations on animals, which Fraenkel had formulated in 1906:

"Are we at all entitled to conclude from the toxic effect of a Digitalis body on the frog's heart on its therapeutic effect on humans?

There were findings indicating different effects of cardiac glycosides in humans and animals. The known but unappreciated contradictions between the results of animal experiments and the observations at the bedside prompted Eden to study *systematically the conditions for effects of Digitalis on sick people.*

In animal experiments on healthy animals it was found that cardiac glycosides in warm-blooded animals lead to an increase in blood pressure and a reduction in heart rate. In order to show this effect, however, dosages had to be chosen which were a multiple of the therapeutic dose in humans. The therapeutic dosages known from the clinic showed no effects in healthy animals. In contrast, clinical experience had shown that cardiac glycosides do not cause an increase in blood pressure in heart patients, but rather a strong reduction in heart rate.

The question *"Why do Digitalis doses, which are completely ineffective in animal experiments, lead to a significant pulse slowdown in sick people without a simultaneous increase in blood pressure?"* could only be answered by examinations on patients. There were no animals suffering from heart disease with clear symptoms. Thus, conditions had to be present in cardiac patients which were missing in animal experiments and explained the divergent reaction of the human body. The clarification of this question should make it possible to identify clinical symptons for whose therapy cardiac glycosides are suitable.

For his studies Eden used *"only the chemically uniform bodies (Strophanthin, Strophoside, Digitoxin, Gitalin-Validogen, Digilanide, Pandigal, Cymarin, Scillars)"*. *"For internal* (oral*) use, Digitalis preparations have become established because the Strophanthus preparations are, at least in part, destroyed in the stomach. Strophanthin has established itself for intravenous application"* [Edens 1944]. He primrily chose Boehringer Mannheim's Kombetin as his preferred Strophanthin preparation.

With exemplary scientific accuracy and unsurpassed certainty in the diagnosis of heart diseases, Edens studied the effect of cardiac glycosides on very different forms of heart diseases. He made intensive use of the newly developed technique of recording and evaluating the electrical activities of the heart muscle fibers as electrocardiogram (ECG). An essential basic knowledge of his studies was that the state of the heart determines the effect of cardiac glycosides.

"This phrase: Changes in the heart itself or, more generally, the state of the organ determines the effect of Digitalis, is the key to all clinical Digitalis problems [Edens 1948].

Edens was able to show that Digitalis glycosides administered orally are particularly effective when the heart is abnormally enlarged (hypertrophy) and is insufficient. Heart glycosides have no effect on healthy hearts, but also on non-insufficient hypertrophic (enlarged) hearts.

Heart failure is not a state that can be clearly defined. There are graded degrees of insufficiency. The concept of insufficiency is only vaguely defined. Particularly in the early stages, insufficiency is a phenomenon that cannot be clearly distinguished. It is often impossible to say where the physiological breathing and pulse acceleration associated with every effort ends and the pathological begins. Accordingly, sliding transitions from full effect to ineffectiveness can also be found in Digitalis. *"Fixed measures and numbers cannot be set up, here the living experience speaks the last word.... The state of the heart thus determines the effect of the Digitalis. And so it also determines the type of application, the size of the dosage, the duration of application."* With this statement, Edens, as Fraenkel had already done, clearly sets himself apart from the request of pharmacologists for standard doses of cardiac glycosides in heart failure.

Every form of cardiac insufficiency reduces the pumping capacity of the heart. The heart pumps less blood, the blood circulation of the body and thus also that of the heart itself decreases. A reduction in heart blood flow leads to weaker heart performance, deepens the insufficiency: a self-reinforcing weakening of the heart begins. This circle must be broken. Cardiac glycosides act on both phases of cardiac activity - filling phase (diastole) and expulsion phase (systole). The effect on the diastole can be seen in the pulse deceleration. The lower the pulse, the longer the filling phase. The effect on the systole can be seen in a faster and stronger contraction of the heart, the pumping volume is increased. Edens was able to show that orally administered Digitalis preparations primarily have a diastolic effect. Strophanthin administered intravenously has a pronounced systolic effect. A difference that Vaquez had already pointed out, but which was denied by Fraenkel.

Systole is crucial for the pumping performance of the heart. Increasing the pumping capacity also promotes blood circulation in the coronary arteries and thus improves cardiac performance. Edens therefore postulated two different effects for cardiac glycosides: an *immediate* and an *indirect* effect. Its *immediate* effect is on diastole and systole, its *indirect* effect is to increase coronary blood flow and increase the capacity and efficiency of cardiac work. The differentiation between the direct and indirect effects of cardiac glycosides also made it possible to understand the often contradictory effects on puls and arrhythmias. Edens has not found any experimental evidence for two different effects of Strophanthin. With this differentiation, he merely tried to explain the improvement of cardiac performance after Strophanthin application. The postulate of the indirect effects of cardiac glycosides is one of Eden's most important findings. It inevitably led him to investigate the effect of Strophanthin on ischemic diseases caused by circulatory disorders - coronary sclerosis, angina pectoris and heart attack. He published his extremely positive results in the treatment of angina pectoris patients with intravenous Strophanthin in 1934, thus justifying the special position of this therapy over oral Digitalis therapy. *"The stimulus of insufficient blood circulation on pathologically irritable coronary arteries is probably the most important cause of angina pectoris and heart attacks. In coronary sclerosis, Strophanthin is the safest and most effective way to eliminate this irritation. It will also be the most effective way to prevent myocardial infarction and, once it has occurred, to counteract its spread and consequences"* [Edens 1944]. For Edens, *"intravenous Strophanthin treatment was the safest treatment for organically induced angina pectoris, including myocardial infarction."* He was convinced that *"The time will come, in which failure to timely start ouabain therapy will be condemned as medical malpractice."*

Ernst Edens laid down his experiences with intravenous Strophanthin therapy - including technical instructions for intravenous injections - in a short *Digitalis booklet* (Digitalisfibel) conceived as a guide for the general practitioner, which was very popular with doctors and was published in several editions [Edens 1944]. A comprehensive scientific presentation is the third version of his Digitalis monograph *Die Digitalisbehandlung* [Edens 1948], published in 1948 - due to the war only four years after his death.

In the *Digitalisfibel*, Edens lists the most important conditions in which intravenously administered Strophanthin is indicated:

- rapid help in case of threatening cardiac failure
- heart failure with slow pulse
- vomiting after oral digitalization
- overstretching of the heart in the final stages of decompensation of valve defects and high pressure
- heart failure without hypertrophy
- coronary sclerosis with cardiac insufficiency, agina pectoris, heart attack
- cardiac insufficiency as a result of myocarditis
- heart failure in arrhythmias as a result of oral digitalisation

It is noteworthy that Edens explicitly points out that Strophanthin eliminates toxic side effects of Digitalis. This observation was already described in 1902 in the literature and has been repeatedly confirmed afterwards. In 2010, David Lichtstein and co-workers again confirmed this effect in in-vitro and in-vivo experiments [Nescher 2010].

A logical consequence of the realization that *the state of the heart determines the effect of Digitalis*, is that from the effect of Digitalis the state of the heart can be concluded. Albert Fraenkel and Ernst Edens have therefore also used Strophanthin therapy for diagnostic purposes. Until well into the 1970s, the Strophanthin test was a common method for diagnosing heart failure[3].

Ernst Edens has always differentiated between *internal* Digitalis - orally administered Digitalis preparations - and *intravenous* Digitalis, Strophanthin. He was convinced that the differences in effects he observed were due to the form of administration and not to differences in the active ingredients. His results met with considerable criticism from many pharmacologically oriented clinicians. These demanded - despite the available successes at the bedside! - an examination in animal experiments. For Edens, this request was proof of a divergence between medicine and pharmacology that Fraenkel also had criticized. Edens appreciated the possibilities of experimental pharmacology, but this should subordinate itself *to clinical thinking, to independent judgment at the patient's bedside. The wellbeing of the sick is the supreme law.* He therefore resisted the request to make the obvious attempt to compare the effect of Strophanthin directly with another Digitalis glycoside in longer observation series: *"Once we have recognized Strophanthin as the best and safest remedy, we no longer have the right to withhold it from a patient, let alone a number of patients, only for scientific reasons, only to test the still uncertain effect of another remedy, and thereby lose a valuable time for healing."*

It was not until 1994 that Italian scientists conducted such a comparative study between intravenous k-Strophanthin and orally administered digoxin in 22 patients with severe heart failure [Agostini 1994]. Strophanthin proved to be superior to digoxin in all measured parameters. The special position of intravenous Strophanthin over other

---

[3] After oral ouabain tablets had become available in the 1950s, the "Strophantine rapid test" enjoyed increasing popularity. Patients with suspected heart disease were given two tablets of 3 mg that they had to chew and distribute in the mouth. In the case of heart disease, a relief of complaints was observed within 5–10 min. This test was used routinely in German physicians' offices well into the 1970s.

cardiac glycosides established by Ernst Edens has been confirmed by the Agostini study.

At the end of the 1930s, intravenous Strophanthin was firmly established as one of the most popular drugs for the treatment of heart diseases in Germany. In his 1947 *textbook on pharmacology,* Fritz Eichholz pays tribute to Fraenkel and Eden's success with intravenous Strophanthin therapy: *"The enormous progress that Strophanthin has brought us results from the statement that almost every physician can keep his decompensated patients free of edema in the wider surroundings of the places of origin of Strophanthin therapy - Heidelberg and Dusseldorf - and usually also ban the horrors of angina pectoris".* Textbooks have highlighted the excellent effects of intravenous Strophanthin. *"The greatest advance in cardiac therapy after Withering is the introduction of Strophanthin."* [Eichholtz 1947]. *"Strophanthin dextrose ampoules containing ouabain are also highly recommended. ... In this form, Strophanthin has proved itself so excellently and has become one of the most popular means of practice"* [Curschmann 1947].

Albert Fraenkel and Ernst Edens have rejected the oral administration of Strophanthin preparations. Both have worked with k-Strophanthin, which is susceptible to hydrolysis and therefore the active ingredient is largely destroyed after oral administration in the stomach. Other authors had reported very positive experiences with oral Strophanthin therapy, especially with the hydrolysis-stable ouabain. However, it was generally accepted that *"Strophanthin administered orally is ineffective. Oral Strophanthin therapy is hardly mentioned in monographs and textbooks because it is considered to be so ineffective that its application or even its verification is unnecessary from the outset."* [Kern 1951].

Info-Box: The heart and its function

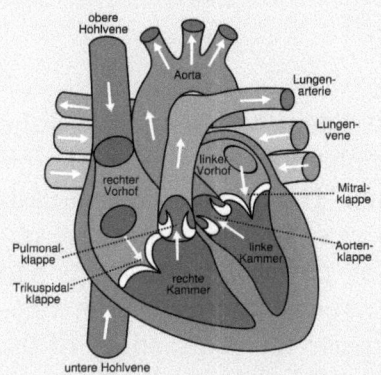

The heart is a hollow muscle with four chambers. The heart septum running along the longitudinal axis of the heart separates the left from the right half of the heart. Each of the two halves of the heart consists of two interiors:

The smaller atria (left and right atrium) collect the blood. The larger chambers (left and right ventricle) suck the blood from the atria and press it into the body or lung circulation. Between the atria and the ventricles, as well as at the openings of the chambers to the large arteries, there are heart valves. The valves ensure that the blood flow always runs in the same direction and prevent the blood from flowing back.

The pumping function of the heart can be divided into two phases: the filling phase (diastole) and the expulsion phase (systole). During the filling phase, the heart relaxes, the chambers are filled with blood: oxygen-rich blood flows from the pulmonary veins into the left atrium, at the same time oxygen-poor blood from the large body veins reaches the right atrium. The blood then flows from the atria into the main chambers, which are filled to about 80 percent of their capacity at the end of the diastole. At a pulse of 60/min the diastole lasts approx. 0.7 seconds. The expulsion phase consists of an atrial systole phase in which both atria contract so that further blood from the atria is forced into the large chambers. This is followed by the expulsion phase (ventricular systole). In this phase, the two main chambers contract. The blood is pressed into the aorta and the pulmonary artery. The entire systole lasts only about 0.3 seconds.

Berthold Kern and Left Failure

Albert Fraenkel, Henri Vaquez and Ernst Edens had investigated the effects of intravenously administered Strophanthin and orally administered Digitalis glycosides in heart patients. The most important indications for the use of cardiac glycosides were known from these clinical studies at the end of the 1940s. The physiological effects had also been determined on the basis of numerous experimental pharmacological studies. Cardiac glycosides increase the contractility of the heart (positive inotropic effect) and are therefore suitable for the treatment of heart failure. They reduce the heart rate (negative chronotropic effect) and the stimulation of conduction speed (negative dromotropic effect). Cardiac glycosides also increase the excitability of the heart muscle (positive bathmotropic effect). These three additional properties justify the use of Digitalis for cardiac arrhythmia and atrial fibrillation.

The decision as to which therapy to use to treat a disease is always influenced by an understanding of the anatomical and physiological conditions underlying the disease. The term *heart failure* only entered medicine in the last quarter of the 19th century. One had learned that dropsy was caused by a heart that was too weak. Oedema was then considered a characteristic of heart failure. The anatomy of the heart with two halves of two chambers each was known. But there was only *one* heart failure. Initial approaches at the beginning of the 20th century to differentiate heart diseases according to anatomical conditions, as Henri Vaquez had done, remained the exception for decades. It was not until the 1930s that a more intensive discussion of the distinction between diseases of the left half of the heart and those of the right half of the heart began. In 1948, the Stuttgart-based internist Berthold Kern presented the first comprehensive differentiation into right- and left-ventrical failure based on scientific findings and strict logic [Kern 1948].

Berthold Kern, born in 1911, studied medicine in Vienna and Königsberg. In 1935 he passed the medical state examination in Freiburg. During the Second World War he worked as a troop doctor on the Eastern Front in Russia and in the military hospital in Ulm. From 1946 to 1990, Kern worked as a physician, internist and cardiologist in his own practice in Stuttgart. In addition to his work in his practice, Kern mainly dealt with cardiological issues, published books and more than 40 special articles. His main interest was the treatment of heart diseases with cardiac glycosides. Berthold Kern died in Stuttgart on October 16, 1995.

On Easter Monday in March 1970, Kern describes in a letter how he came to deal with fundamental questions of medicine. His thinking was, as he writes, influenced by Greek philosophy:

"One of the prerequisites for (my) findings is probably that my thinking structure may be somewhat different than usual. My thinking has always been eminently visual; not directly so visual that I could always draw what I saw; but in quasi-spatial relationships of an abstract kind, in which the forces of effect and, strangely enough, the logical connections of nature also appear before the spiritual eye and make their energetic, temporal, causal, logical functional relationships visible in spatio-temporal execution. Even as a schoolboy I saw the pulling forces on the lever arm in this way, how they pull differently depending on the distance from the pivot point, I saw how the electrons scurry through the wire and act outwards; later I saw how the stronger of the two hearts with the congestion pressure presses the blood into the insufficient heart and thus pumps its force up; I have seen how the edema starts up and becomes a prerequisite for the congestion pressure, how this compensatory structure collapses with edema abortion and the heart has to fail; I have seen how the left inner layers are rhythmically white-pressed and thus rhythmically blocked with their metabolism inflow and outflow and suffer from it. ..."

It was only much later that I learned that even the ancient Greeks had shaped the happy word of *gnómes ópsis* for this kind of intellectual (intellectual-abstract) perceptiveness.... The *gnómes ópsis* grasps not only the facts, but also their relationships, their functions, and thus also their "logic" in the broadest sense of the word, for which we have to develop our "methodological logic" for comprehension."

Berthold Kern always sought to classify individual facts as part of a logical whole. He searched for *the creative forces and laws that underlie the superficially visible diseases in the depths.* He attached great importance to pathogenesis *because it is only in pathogenesis that the invisible forces of action that allow the disease patterns to emerge from the causes of the disease are revealed.* Kern regarded medicine as a natural science for which *a consciously trained, constantly strict concept and language breeding* was *indispensable. This* was a demand that had not yet been met in many areas of medicine. In many cases, knowledge gaps were (and are) filled with spongy descriptions - "nervous heart complaints", "heart neurosis", "organ neurosis" - or other terms - "cardiovascular decompensation", "cardiovascular insufficiency", "dilatation" - simply ambiguously used out of habit and carelessness. For Kern, scientific progress in medicine could only result from critical observation of nature and inductive thinking: the summary of unprejudicedly observed details of general laws from which new findings can be logically derived.

During his studies Berthold Kern wrote scripts for a total of 14 subjects. The *blessed compulsion to systematics, classification, logical and didactic order of the material, which lies in such script writing,* was relatively easy for him, as he writes. A publisher he knew planned to publish "Learning Books of Medicine" after the war and commissioned Kern to write the internal medicine volume. Just released from captivity, unemployed, the practice not yet opened, Kern accepted the offer. While writing, he became aware that medical practice and its customary presentation in important areas of medicine not only differed from one another, but often even stood in opposition to one another. In an effort to clarify contradictions, Kern often preceded his corresponding treatises with definitions of terms. Kern's book *Grundlagen der Inneren Medizin*, which he wrote together with his wife Margarete Kern, was published by Enke Verlag in 1946. Kern was particularly interested in the chapter on heart diseases. He expanded this into a monograph, which appeared in 1948 under the title *Die Herzinsuffizienz*. Based on the known facts, he describes a logical picture of heart failure, its manifestations and therapeutic options.

The central phenomenon is contraction failure, which is caused by damage to the heart muscle (myogenic insufficiency) or chronic overload (ergogenic insufficiency). Kern was convinced that myogenic insufficiency is not only caused by a lack of oxygen in the heart muscle. He suspects that, among other factors, cardiac metabolic disorders may also be involved. This assumption was later transferred to the pathogenesis of myocardial infarction.

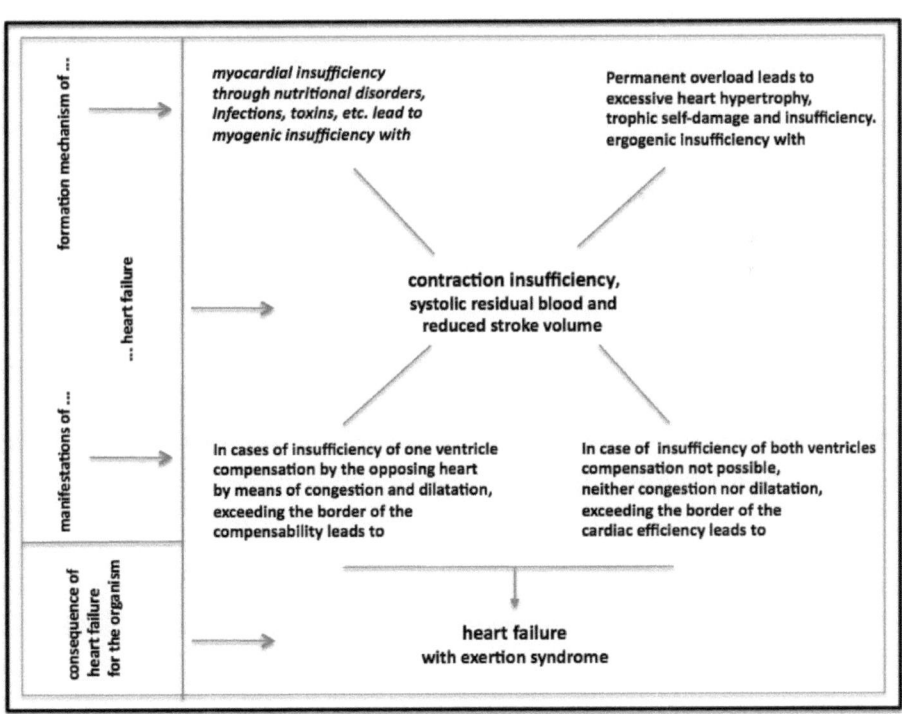

Kern differentiates between right- and left-ventricle failure in the manifestations of heart failure. In left-ventricle failure, in addition to the
standard symptom of reduced performance (exertion syndrome), sleep
disorders are particularly frequent and are a serious indication of the
onset of heart failure. This observation is confirmed by current
research results. In 2014, Norwegian scientists published the results
of a large-scale observational study of 70,000 adults. Patients with
severe sleep disturbances (sleep disturbance, sleep-through disturbance and no nightly recovery) fall ill with heart failure much more
frequently than patients without sleep disturbances. The researchers
conclude that sleep disorders are an important indication of a cardiovascular risk [Laugsand 2014].

Right-ventrical failure with its congestions in the large circuit is the
reservoir for all severe heart failures that have to be treated in
hospital. Therefore, clinicians at university clinics and hospitals were
particularly familiar with this form of heart failure. Patients with left-
ventrical failure were rarely seen by the clinicians in hospitals. This
patient pool was treated by practitioners. For university physicians,
therefore, there was only *one* heart failure. Correspondingly great was
the skepticism with which Kern's depictions were taken up. Today,
many of the descriptions in Kern's monograph *Die Herzinsuffizienz*
(Heart Failure) belong to the general knowledge in medicine.

As a physician in private practice, Berthold Kern was an outsider for
university cardiologists who was not believed to contribute fundamental knowledge of his own to cardiology. One of the frequently
asked questions was: *"From whom did you get this?"* or as Curschmann put it: *"I have often asked myself, where did the colleague, who
as a student and intern got to know our clinical treatment methods in
detail, after a few years produce his very different and strange
theory?"* [Curschmann 1947]. When Kern began to transform his
theoretical findings into practical applications two years later, amused
scepticism soon turned into an aggressive rejection of his theory of
heart failure.

	left insufficiency . . .	right insufficiency . . .	double insufficiency . . .
... with sufficient circulation	congestion all over small circuit with right hypertrophy and left dilatation; congestion lung, possibly to the "pulmonary edema"; neurogenic dyspnoea, possibly cardiac asthma, nyktopnoe; decrease in (systolic) blood pressure. especially in hypertonic patients. insufficiency stenocardias	congestion all over large circuit with left hypertrophy and right dilatation; swelling of the liver and other organs; stasis cyanosis and cardiac edema, nycturia; Rise of the (diast.) Blood pressure, possibly also congestive hypertension frequent atrial fibrillation	externally no repercussions and symptons
... with insufficient circulation	the same, in addition exertion syndrome	the same, in addition exertion syndrome	exertion syndrome

Kern recommended cardiac glycosides for the drug therapy of heart failure. For him, they were *the* heart failure treatment par excellence. It was known that heart extracts can increase the performance of insufficient hearts.[4] Kern deduced the hypothesis that there is one (or more) *heart fuel(s)* that are essential for the conversion of chemical energy into mechanical energy. Although the muscle-chemical mode of action is still little researched, *cardiac glycosides are believed to act in the sense of substituting a substance missing in cardiac insufficiency, which might be chemically closely related to them.*

Of the numerous species of cardiac glycosides from the animal and plant kingdom, only Strophanthus and Digitalis glycosides were considered for therapeutic use:

"The best cardiac glycoside is Strophanthin: it has the most intensive therapeutic effect and almost no toxic side effects. ... Its only disadvantage is the need for intravenous administrati-

---

[4] The effects of heart extracts *(corhormone)* have indeed been the subject of intensive research for decades.

on, which often limits or excludes its use outside the hospital. ... Digitalis glycosides have a less favorable effect. They must be administered in much larger quantities until their therapeutic effect is equal to that of Strophanthin, but their toxic side effects increase in at least the same proportion. In the damaged myocardium, so in all myogenic and all severe insufficiencies, the toxic phenomena occur particularly early and strongly and can even in tiny doses exceed the therapeutic effect, so that the heart is worse off with Digitalis than without them..... The only advantage of Digitalis glycosides is the possibility of oral or rectal administration." [Kern 1948]

This assessment of Digitalis glycosides - formulated in November 1947! - is shared by all cardiologists today. It corresponds to the current state of science and is the reason why Digitalis glycosides are only secondary in the guidelines for the treatment of heart failure.

Info Box: Heart Failure

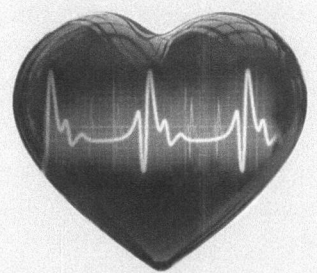

Heart failure is the result of diseases that prevent the heart from maintaining the body's blood circulation. The older you get, the higher the risk of heart failure. In people aged 65 to 75, two to five percent suffer from heart failure, in people aged 70 to 80 this figure is 10 to 20 percent. The prognosis is very unfavorable. Overall, half of the patients die within four years. Of the patients who have been hospitalized for heart failure, 40 percent die or are hospitalized again in one year. Heart failure is one of the most common causes of death. The mortality rate is similar to that of cancer.

Diseases that cause heart failure:

- Coronary Artery Disease (CAD): CAD causes deposits in the coronary arteries. According to textbook interpretation, this can limit the supply of the heart muscles under stress. Heart pain and tightness in the chest (angina pectoris) can occur. In the narrowed blood vessel sections, a blood clot can completely close a coronary vessel and thus trigger an acute heart attack. CAD is the most common cause of heart failure.

- heart attack as a result of coronary heart disease

- hypertension

- heart valve defect

- myocarditis

- heart muscle diseases (cardiomyopathies)

- cardiac arrhythmia

Heart failure develops gradually over months or years. For a long time, the body succeeds in compensating for cardiac insufficiency through faster heartbeat, enlargement of the heart muscle (hypertrophy) and narrowing of the blood vessels. If this compensation is successful, it is called *compensated* heart failure. Symptoms only occur during physical exertion. If compensation is no longer possible, decompensated heart failure occurs. Symptoms already occur at rest or under low stress. Pathological accumulation of water in the tissue (edema) and shortness of breath occur.

The symptoms that can occur with heart failure are many and varied. The main symptom is shortness of breath, which initially only occurs during physical exertion, later also at rest. Added to this are:

- tiredness and listlessness

- severe insomnia (difficulty falling asleep, difficulty sleeping through, breathing difficulties)

- swollen legs and feet

- swollen or taut stomach, loss of appetite

- increased urination at night

- confusion, memory problems

- cough with "foamy" sputum

Which symptoms occur depends on which ventricle is affected and whether only one or both ventricles are affected. In right heart failure, increased pressure in the lungs due to illness leads to a backlog in the blood flow. Blood congests in the incoming veins. The right ventricle must then pump the blood into the lungs with more force. The heart is overloaded and damaged. The increased pressure in the veins causes water to accumulate in the body, especially in the legs and abdomen. Right heart failure usually develops as a result of chronic left heart failure.

In left heart failure, the pumping capacity of the left half of the heart is no longer sufficient. the blood is retained in the pulmonary vessels. Coughing and shortness of breath are typical symptoms.

Heart failure is usually classified according to the severity of its symptoms. The New York Heart Association divides heart failure into classes I, II, III and IV.

Class I: no symptoms - The patient feels no symptoms, is neither short of breath nor fatigued during physical activity.

Class II: Mild heart failure - The patient is short of breath or exhausted after moderate activity.

Class III: Moderate to severe heart failure - The patient is short of breath or exhausted after low activity.

Class IV: Severe heart failure - The patient is exhausted, short of breath and tired, even when sitting still or lying in bed.

Calcification of the coronary arteries (coronary artery disease) is considered the most common cause of heart failure. This calcification of the vessels constrict blood supply to the heart muscle. As a result, the heart muscle is undersupplied and is no longer efficient. The second main cause is high blood pressure (hypertension). If you have high blood pressure, your heart needs to pump more strongly for a long time. However, it will not withstand this strain for a long time - the pumping capacity is declining. Other causes are cardiac arrhythmia, myocarditis and heart valve defects.

Medicinal therapy:

Active ingredients from the group of ACE inhibitors, beta-blockers and diuretics are used as standard.

ACE inhibitors lower blood pressure and thus relieve the heart. If ACE inhibitors are not tolerated, AT1 antagonists are used. These block the effect of a blood pressure-increasing hormone and thus lower the blood pressure.

Beta-blockers prevent cardiac arrhythmia and improve the prognosis of heart failure.

Diuretics are diuretic drugs. They excrete stored liquid and thus reduce the strain on the heart and blood vessels.

If necessary, active ingredients from other substance classes are also used.

Digitalis preparations are only used as "reserve drugs" if the other drugs alone are no longer sufficient. An exception is the recommended use for frequency control in atrial fibrillation, a common form of cardiac arrhythmia.

Oral Strophanthin treatment

In his monograh *Grundlagen der Inneren Medizin* (foundations of internal medicine) Berthold Kern has attempted to present logical descriptions of diseases and the resulting conclusions based on an analysis of physicians experiences and scientific findings. In the book *Die Herzinsuffizienz* (Heart Failure) he has further deepened this procedure of *historical analysis* as he called it, for heart failure. The subject of the analysis was the disease with all its causes and manifestations. The therapy of heart failure was not the focus of attention. Kern only came across very contradictory reports of experiences with oral Strophanthin in the treatment of heart patients when he was working on *Die Herzinsuffizienz*. In his previous books he had adopted the doctrine valid in the 1940s that orally administered Strophanthin was ineffective. In contrast to Digitalis preparations, Strophanthin must be administered intravenously. How could it be then that John Kirk had already felt a fast and clear slowing down of his pulse by minimal contact with Strophanthus poison arrows while brushing his teeth? Hadn't Fraser been able to achieve numerous successes in his treatments of patients with Strophanthus tincture, which led him to the conviction that Strophanthus was superior to Digitalis? Were all the positive results with the numerous oral Strophanthus preparations available on the market all just the result of charlatanism and imagination? If the dogma of the oral ineffectiveness of Strophanthin were unreservedly true, Strophanthin could not have been discovered.

The very beneficial therapeutic effects of intravenous Stropanthin[5] were generally accepted. Fraenkel, Edens, Vaquez and others had shown that it was superior to Digitalis preparations. The risk of

---

[5] Until the 1950s, it was rarely differentiated between k-Strophanthin and g-Strophanthin (ouabain) due to consistent effects. Many older works do not show which Strophanthin was used, only the use of "Strophanthin" is reported.

Strophanthin death due to improper dosage was considered manageable. The doctors often expressed the desire for an oral preparation that was also suitable for the outpatient treatment of heart failure. This would also meet Fraenkel's and Eden's request for early Strophanthin prophylaxis in heart failure. Kern analysed the published very variable experiences with orally administered cardiac glycosides. He identified several problem areas that had led to the prevailing doctrine. Two were of particular importance: the quality of the preparations and an assessment of the glycoside effects and thus also of the preparations, which changed under the influence of experimental pharmacology.

The quality of the preparations, long a serious problem with Strophanthus and Digitalis preparations, had increased significantly with the availability of pure active ingredients. However, it was noticeable that some doctors, as well as Fraenkel, observed that tinctures can be advantageous over pure substances. Kern describes his own observation on the phenomenon of the uncertain effect of Strophanthus preparations, the implications of which neither he himself nor generations of critics of oral Strophanthin therapy have become aware of:

> *"And we ourselves can also confirm from our numerous preliminary tests that not only different Strophanthins and Strophanthin mixtures, but also the same glycoside in the same dosage and application can have a strong effect on the same person, depending on the nature of the indifferent vehicle itself, but can also have little or no effect."* [Kern 1951, p. 17].

The significant influence of galenics on the effect of cardiac glycosides, the *influence of the indifferent vehicle*, only became the focus of scientific attention 30 years later in the 1980s, when systematic galenical research began. For Kern, fluctuating qualities of the preparations were not a fundamental problem. Since Withering, general practitioners have been accustomed to dosing cardiac glycosides individually according to the patient's needs. This procedure was in accordance with Eden's rule *"Every heart has its own Digitalis dose."* Different potencies could therefore be easily compensated by adjusting the dosage. In addition, Strophanthin had a decisive advantage over Digitalis: when administered orally, fatal poisoning was ruled out. The side effects of too high doses were limited to diarrhoea and vomiting, some of them very severe. There were no reports of oral Strophanthin deaths. This is not the case with oral Digitalis, where there have been numerous deaths, as reported already by Withering.

More problematic than the potency of Strophanthus preparations were the assessments of glycoside effects by pharmacology. The pharmacology of the Schmiedeberg School was dedicated to study toxic effects of substances on healthy animals. Albert Fraenkel had named the resulting fundamental problem: *"Are we at all entitled to conclude from the toxic effect of a Digitalis body on the frog's heart on its therapeutic effect on humans?"* Ernst Edens, a physician such as Albert Fraenkel, had expressly denied this question and pleaded for a *"systematic investigation of the conditions of effect of Digitalis on sick people"*. Schmiedeberg, on the other hand, was convinced that an experiment on healthy animals *"would enable him to determine with certainty whether a substance promises beneficial success as a drug."* This claim was in clear contradiction to medical experience. A contradiction which was clearly formulated by many doctors and clinicians. However, the supposed superiority of scientifically objective measurement on animals or isolated animal organs prevailed over the subjective observations of physicians at the bedside. Remedies and poison became synonyms. Paracelsus' saying *"All things are poison, and nothing is without poison; only the dose makes that a thing is not poison"* became the guideline of pharmacology. H. H. Meyer therefore spoke in his *textbook of pharmacology as the basis of drug treatment* in 1936 no longer of drugs, but only of poisons. In his 1947 *textbook on pharmacology*, Fritz Eichholtz confessed: *"Pharmacology - like all other theoretical subjects of medicine - has rather detached itself from the clinic because the enormous tasks that lay before it could no longer be solved by observation on humans, but only by animal experiments."*

In his third book, *Die orale Strophanthin Behandlung* (oral Strophan-thin treatment) Berthold Kern describes the consequences of this alie-nation of the *scientific* pharmacology of cardiac glycosides from me-dical practice [Kern 1951]. All cardiac glycosides, whether derived from Digitalis or Strophanthus species, cause cardiac death in animals if sufficient doses are applied. The lethal dose of the individual active ingredients varies. This observation led to Schmiedeberg's conclusi-on, praised by Fraenkel as a *great deed,* that the cardiac glycosides all have the same qualitative effect and differ only in the quantity of their effect. To determine the potency of cardiac glycoside preparations, it had become common practice to determine the intravenous dose le-thal to frogs and to state it as *frog-unit.* It was known from the clinic that the full effect of Digitalis preparations on patients could only be observed after a few days. The effect of Strophanthus preparations, on the other hand, was felt after just a few minutes. Corresponding diffe-rences were found in the determination of the potency in animals, which had the unpleasant disadvantage that the determination of Digi-talis preparations was more time-consuming than that of Strophan-thins. Therefore, the potency determination was modified to a quick test. This method, introduced by Straub in 1916, became the officially prescribed standard method in Germany in 1928 for obtaining phar-macological assessments on cardiac glycosides. In this *timeless* rapid test, the glycosides were applied so quickly and in such high doses that the animal died within four hours. While the lethal effect of the usual low doses of Strophanthus preparations was also very rapid in this test, very high doses had to be selected for the Digitalis prepara-tions. These were orders of magnitude higher than the doses known to humans from hospitals. Schmiedeberg had considered Strophanthin to be insufficiently effective, i.e. too little toxic - and therefore warned Krehl to approve Fraenkel's experiments with Strophanthin in pati-ents - but Strophanthin was now scientifically proven to be the most toxic of all glycosides. The rapid test had made Digitoxin, which has been clinically extremely toxic since Withering, the least toxic cardi-ac glycoside. This *scientifically exactly* determined toxicity of Strophanthin apparently correlated with the *Strophantin death* observed with too high doses in intravenous application. This strengthened Strophanthin's reputation as dangerous and unpredictable.

The slow onset effect of the active ingredients of Digitalis was in principle a disadvantage in practice compared to the fast-acting active ingredients of Strophanthus. In an effort to shorten the long latency time and thus better control the effect, the dubious methodological approach of the timeless rapid test of compensating for slow onset effects by high doses was transferred to clinical practice. Contrary to Withering's justification of the ascending dosing of Digitalis, a *Digitalisstoss* (Digitalis push) was recommended. Treatment started with a high dose. The full dose (understood as the maximum effect on the heart, judged by the slowing down of the heart rate) should be administered as quickly as possible. The subsequent doses were then successively reduced (maintenance dose). This dosage scheme developed in the USA became popular in Germany after 1945 and contributed significantly to the fact that Digitalis poisoning was the most frequent poisoning by drugs in Germany in the post-war period.

Kern drew attention to the methodological errors of the experimental pharmacological assessment of cardiac glycosides. The therapeutic value of an active substance cannot be derived solely from its toxicity. What is decisive is the relationship between therapeutic effect and toxic side effects, which Kern defined as the *efficacy quotient*. Today, the terms *therapeutic width* and *therapeutic window* are used for this. An active substance with high toxicity can also have a very wide therapeutic range if the therapeutic effect is achieved at doses far below the dose at which the toxic effects occur. Likewise, a substance which is toxic only in high doses has a small therapeutic window if the dosage required for the therapeutic effect is comparable to the toxic dose. Today we know that Digitalis drugs have a very narrow therapeutic range. Even within the therapeutic range toxic side effects are possible.

Despite the methodological misconceptions, there was a clear discrepancy between the measurements of experimental pharmacology and the medical experience with oral Strophanthin. Oral administration of

Strophanthus preparations required much higher doses than intravenous administration. Intravenously 0.25 - 0.5 mg per day were considered as optimal, orally the doses were up to 30 mg without symptoms of poisoning. Digitalis preparations could also only be administered orally in doses of a few milligrams per day in order to avoid poisoning. However, since the pharmacological rapid test had determined Strophanthin as very toxic and the Digitalis active substances as relatively non-toxic, this obvious contradiction between pharmacology and clinic had to be explained. The high hydrolysis sensitivity of k-Strophanthin was known. The high doses required for oral administration of Strophanthin were therefore interpreted as hydrolysis of the active substance in the gastrointestinal tract. The g-Strophanthin (ouabain) is hydrolysis stable. Therefore, a low absorption was assumed as an alternative. The active ingredient would be excreted undecomposed.

The measurement results of experimental pharmacology and their interpretation soon found their way into textbooks. That is why Kern writes at the end of the 1940s that oral Strophanthin therapy was *hardly mentioned* in monographs and textbooks *because, according to unanimous opinion, it is so ineffective that its application or even its verification is unnecessary from the outset.*

Strophoral

"We have an injustice to make amends for." With this admission Berthold Kern begins his book *Die orale Strophanthin-Behandlung* [Kern 1951]. He no longer wanted to limit himself to theoretical analyses and explanations. He was convinced: *"The best cardiac glycoside is Strophanthin: it has the most intensive therapeutic effect and almost no toxic side effects"*. The restriction to intravenous application was based on methodologically questionable measurements and prejudices. Although there were still some oral Strophanthin products such as the Purostrophan from Kali Chemie, these led a shadowy existence. Digitalis products dominated the market for heart failure. Kern's goal was to revive oral Strophanthin therapy.

Industry was also very interested in Kern's comments on the special role of Strophanthin in the treatment of heart failure. Sandoz from Basel and Boehringer Mannheim sought dialogue. A special meeting of the Boehringers scientific committee was held in Mannheim to define the further strategy for Strophanthin. An oral Strophanthin was considered a good supplement to Kombetin. In April 1948, Dr. Rabald, Head of Research at Boehringer, visited Kern several times. They agreed on cooperation. As early as June 1948, Boehringer produced Strophantin tablets on an experimental basis, according to Kern's suggestions. In July, Strophanthin lozenges for perlingual application were added to the test series. Kern tested the Boehringer tablets on selected patients and was delighted. The first two patients were a complete therapeutic success. Because of the known risk of side effects at doses of more than 0.5 mg iv per day, Boehringer had adjusted the tablets to an active substance content of 0.25 mg. The fear of Strophantin death was omnipresent. However, more than 10 tablets per day were needed to achieve a safe effect. The active substance content was then increased to 3 mg per tablet. In December 1948, the cooperation partners decided to develop a lozenge. Boehringer provided Kern with Strophanthin tablets made from various Strophanthus active ingredients and mixtures from which the *noble mixture* was to be selected. While Kern was still testing the various Strophanthins, Boehringer was discussing internally whether the company should dare to offer a product from which according to prevailing doctrine no therapy and thus no commercial success could be expected. Boehringer also had the preparations tested by other doctors. Finally it was agreed to take the risk.

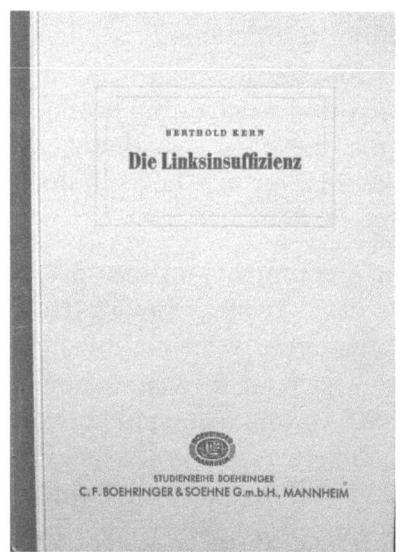

Die Linksinsuffizienz published by Boehringer Mannheim for the promotion of *Strophoral*

The active ingredient was ouabain, to which a small percentage of k-Strophanthin chemically modified by hydrogenation was added. The preparation was adjusted as a lozenge for perlingual application. Information on the galenic composition of the tablets is not known. The commercial management of the company asked Kern for a memorandum with which sceptical doctors and clinicians could be convinced of the advantages of oral Strophanthin therapy. The date for the launch of the *Strophoral* baptized preparation was set for July 1, 1949 and was also adhered to. A few months later, a Strophoral solution was also offered. Boehringer distributed a Strophoral advertising brochure to 30,000 doctors, with an attached order card for free samples and for a booklet written by Kern entitled *Die Linksinsuffizienz*. It presented Kern's views on left-ventricle failure and the therapeutic successes achieved with Strophoral. Kern also published an article in the *Deutsche Medizinische Wochenschrift* entitled "Strophoral - Zur Erneuerung der oralen Strophanthustherapie" (Strophoral - The Renewal of Oral

74

Strophanthus Therapy) [Kern 1949]. On January 5, 1950, his 39th birthday, Berthold Kern and Boehringer Mannheim signed a cooperation agreement. The agreement guaranteed Kern remuneration for his cooperation in the form of a share in sales.

Strophoral sales significantly exceeded Boehringer's expectations. Production bottlenecks occurred. There was a lack of packaging material. Glass vials had to be used in place of the intended tin cans. By October 1949 alone, more than 15,000 copies of the *Linksinsuffizienz* booklet had been requested. The feedback from general practitioners was predominantly positive. Quite often there were indications of irritations and inflammations in the mouth area, which soon were controled by correcting the tablet formulation. More serious was the criticism from university clinicians who told Boehringer in letters that they had fallen for *unproven stuff from a provincial practitioner*. In a crisis meeting with Kern it was decided not to rush things too quickly, to react cautiously and not to provoke any further resistance, after all *business is going well beyond expectations*. But the resistance from the ranks of the university chairs grew. Boros published a devastating assessment under the title "Strophoral - a therapeutic error" [Boros 1951]. The Stuttgart clinician Beckmann was quoted by Boehringer as saying, *"I have never seen what Kern calls left-ventricle failure, and what he calls double failure does not even exist."* The feedback from general practitioners continued to be predominantly positive. But Boehringer feared for its reputation among university clinicians.

In September 1950, research director Rabald travelled to Kern in Stuttgart and tried to dissuade him from publishing his monograph on oral Strophanthin treatment, which was about to be completed. Kern resisted. A crisis meeting was held in Mannheim on October 7. Boehringer insisted on separating the question of the effectiveness of Strophoral from Kern's theory of heart failure. The general practitioners were not interested in a theoretical dispute. Therefore, Kern should refrain from publishing his Strophoral Monograph or at least wait until the excitement has settled around the theory of heart failure. Kern adhered to his plans to publish the book. In the following months, the dispute between Kern and Boehringer intensified. Lawyers have been called in. Individual chapters in the manuscript of the book were discussed. Boehringer insisted that Kern makes it clear in the book that its content does not represent Boehringer's views. The book [Kern 1951] was published in May 1951. Kern emphasized, as requested by Boehringer, that Boehringer does not share his views: *"As requested, we emphasize that the main contents of this book - the reasons and the initiative for the renewal of oral Strophanthin treatment, the development of theoretical and practical methods, prerequisites, results, conclusions, etc. are not shared by Boehringer but are independent scientific achievements of the author, from no side materially, by suggestions, literature procurement or otherwise supported, rather under victims against various handicaps compiled, and that the opinions of the company C. F. Boehringer and sons deviate in substantial points from our results".* (Kern 1951, p. 94].

In November 1950 Berthold Kern received a visit from a colleague, Dr. Peter Mutschler, general practitioner in Offenau near Heilbronn. Mutschler reported about interesting experiences with modified Strophoral tablets. He had covered them with an enteric varnish that causes the tablets to dissolve only in the small intestine and release the active ingredient there. These tablets, which he called *duodenal tablets*, had already shown good therapeutic success at significantly lower doses than the usual Strophoral dosage. Mutschler had submitted his results to Boehringer in October 1950 and asked for cooperation, but received no response from Mannheim. He asked Kern for support for his project and for intercession at Boehringer. On February 17, 1951, Kern and Mutschler signed an agreement on joint efforts to develop duodenal Strophanthin products. On May 20, they extended this agreement to all drugs *which serve cardiac therapy.* The contract assured each partner of 50 percent of any income. Kern committed himself in the contract to support Mutschler's project at Boehringer. Mutschler undertook to present his process to other companies.

Kern contacted Rabald, who led Boehringer to produce various enteric coated tablets and have them tested by pharmacologists and clinicians. On February 14, 1951, Boehringer announced to Mutschler that Boehringer had no interest in the development of duodenal Strophoral. Kern derived from his contract with Boehringer that Boehringer was obliged to implement his proposals, i.e. to promote the duodenal Strophoral project. The dispute with Boehringer escalated. Finally, Boehringer terminated the contract with Kern on January 1, 1952, resulting in severe financial losses for Kern. Long-drawn-out legal disputes followed. Kern was unable to assert any claims against Boehringer.

Boehringer Mannheim marketed the oral Strophoral preparations until the 1970s. Approvals officially expired on April 30,1990.

After Boehringer had decided not to develop a duodenal Strophanthin preparation, Mutschler contacted to Kali-Chemie. It had already marketed an ouabain solution, Purostrophan, for both intravenous and oral therapy. *Purostrophan drops liquidum* had been sold since 1904. Shortly thereafter, a *Purostrophan injection solution* was added. Rudolf Franck had described Purostrophan in his handbook *Modern Therapy in Internal Medicine and General Practice* 1943 *"to have a favorable effect on perlingual application"* [Franck 1943].

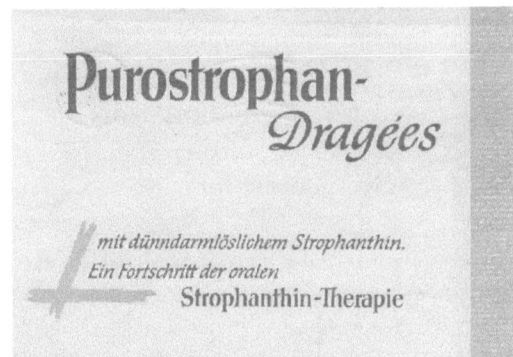

Advertising motif of Kali-Chemie

Based on the preliminary work of Mutschler Kali-Chemie developed Dragées, which were coated with an enteric lacquer. In January 1953 the product was offered under the name *Purostrophan Dragées*. Mutschler received a contractually guaranteed remuneration in the form of a revenue share. Kali-Chemie had the dragées tested by university clinicians and pharmacologists during their development. However, these were only willing to cooperate with the written assurance from Kali-Chemie that the product development was not related to *Kern's cardiology*. In a letter to Kern, dated January 29, 1953, Mutschler listed a number of professors who had insisted on such a distancing. Kali-Chemie protested against any contact with Kern. When Mutschler prepared a publication on the use of Purostrophan Dragées in combination with other preparations, Mutschler was asked to make *"some changes in the text, by which the reference to Kern's works is dispensed with"*. The rejection of Kern's theory of heart failure by university chairs was massive. Kali-Chemie could not resist this either. The cooperation between Mutschler and Kern became more and more difficult due to the resulting tensions and ended in a dispute.

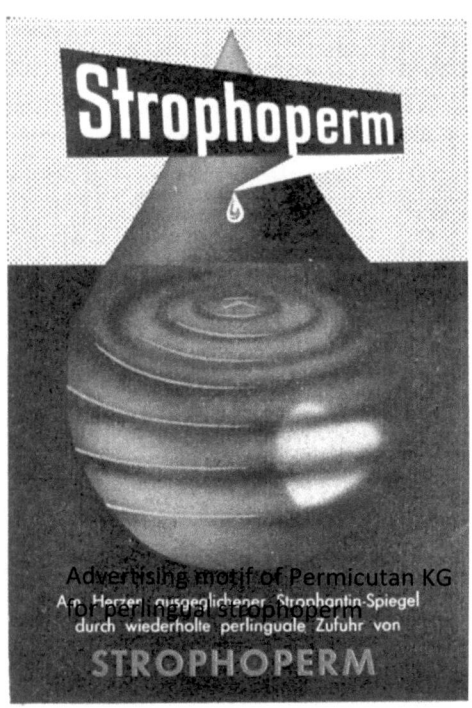

Advertising motif of Permicutan KG

PERMICUTAN-KG · DR. EULER · MÜNCHEN 13

In the 1950s and 1960s, numerous other oral Strophanthin preparations were marketed by various companies. In addition to Strophoral and Purstrophan, optimized preparations for perlingual application (Strophoperm, Strodival) and enteric forms (Strodival MR, Alvonal MR) were particularly successful. The Alvonal MR of Diwag, Berlin, contained the active ingredient Cymarin (k-Strophanthin-α) [Lampe 1968, Krämer 1972]. This is characterized by a significantly higher inherent bioavailability compared to ouabain. The same applies to *Convacard*. This contained the active ingredient Convallatoxin, which is found in lilies of the valley (Convallaria majalis) and whose structure is similar to that of Cymarin (strophanthidin-l-rhamnoside).

On June 28, 1967, the managing director of Permicutan KG, which introduced Strophoperm in 1949, describes in a letter to a friend his experiences as a manufacturer of an oral Strophanthin preparation:

"It has not been one of the joys of life in the last 18 years to carry and sell a Strophanthin preparation yourself. Right from the start, the clinicians dismissed oral Strophanthin preparations as ineffective and made the general practitioners reluctant to prescribe them. Towards the end of the 1950s, Digitalis therapy was largely adopted from Anglo-Saxon countries and, in contrast, Strophanthin was largely postponed. For Strophoperm, however, there have remained loyal prescribers who have been convinced of the benefits of the preparation and its effects for many years. Apparently many hospitals even use Strophoperm without wanting to admit it to the outside world, because we have a disproportionately high sales volume in hospital packages.

Since about 10 years the trade with Semen Strophanthi, the raw material for the production of pure g-Strophanthin, has fallen into uncontrollable hands. Allegedly, thanks to the abundant development aid, the Negroes are no longer supposed to go into the jungle to collect Semen Strophanthi, so that there was a great shortage and increase in price on the world market. Suddenly there was no Strophanthin to find. The scarce quantities that were still available were traded at 10 - 20 times the price. Then the product was once again available at short notice, abundant and inexpensive, in order to disappear from the market just as quickly. ... Experts were of the opinion that on the world market a rocking policy was being pursued at our expense, which ultimately helped to push back Strophanthin in favour of other cardiac drugs".

Oral Strophanthin preparations have always remained niche products in comparison to the Digitalis preparations used on a large scale.

The Strophoral Dispute

Boehringer Mannheim made every effort to defuse the scientific dispute over Strophoral. While Berthold Kern fought primarily for recognition of his theory of heart failure, Boehringer was keen to highlight the practical successes in various indications beyond all theory. At the end of 1951, a brochure entitled *"Für und Wider die orale Strophanthintherapie"* (Pro and Con of oral Strophanthin Therapy) was published that was no longer coordinated with Kern. All clinical and pharmacological publications on the oral use of ouabain that had become known until then are listed in chronological order of their contents. The preface to the brochure says:

> "When we decided about two years ago to supplement our product range for Strophanthin, which previously contained Kombetin for intravenous application, Myocombin for intramuscular administration, and Kombetin suppositories, with an oral Strophanthin preparation, we followed numerous and very emphatic requests from the medical practice, while relinquishing certain concerns. We were of the opinion that we should also make such a preparation, as it is often used at home and abroad, available within the scope of our proven cardiac drug program.
>
> We were surprised to discover shortly after its introduction that interest in such a preparation was unusually high.
>
> But we were even more surprised by the literary echo of the preparation in pharmacological and clinical literature. There was talk of a "Strophoral dispute."

Kern's work is also listed in the brochure and commented objectively and neutrally:

"The author, who at the beginning had probably interpreted the indications for oral Strophanthin much more broadly than other examiners, combined with his observations from outpatient practice a special cardiological theory, which cannot be presented here in its entirety.

He argues that in addition to classical heart failure, there are a large number of patients with latent failure and predominantly subjective complaints. He describes this type of disease as "left ventricle failure" and believes that it accounts for 95% of all heart patients, so that the usual clinical observations about the effect of cardiac glycosides refer only to a very limited number of the actually present heart patients.

The author's successes therefore refer primarily to these latent "left-failures", but also show that even severe edematous heart insufficiencies can be successfully treated with oral Strophanthin. However, the doses must then be considerably increased.

The success stories and cardiological doctrines linked here must be discussed independently of each other."

The commercial success of Strophoral proved a high acceptance of the product by general practitioners. Heilmeyer quoted an internist with a large practice: *"Oral Strophoral therapy is one of the most epoch-making treatments published in many years. It is hard to put into words what joy and salvation this means for my heart patients and for me."* [Heilmeyer 1952]. Positive results were also reported from other clinics [Altmann 1952]. On the other hand, there were publications on the total ineffectiveness of the preparation. These very different clinical experiences with Strophoral were overlaid by the rejection of Kern's theory of heart failure by university clinicians. *"Many renowned cardiologists have already described the symptoms of left-ventricle failure in detail, excellently and in many cases. It was not necessary for Kern to rediscover left-ventricle failure."* Boros [1951]. The only recognized form of heart failure was the variant associated with congestion and edema, which Kern described as *right-ventricle failure*. The disease symptons described by Kern as left-ventricle failure were not accepted as heart diseases. Heilmeyer took the view that cases that respond well to Strophoral are not muscle-damaged hearts, but *"dysregulations of the circulation, in which an unclarified Strophoral effect might have a favourable effect"* [Heilmeyer 1952]. In a review of the book *Die orale Strophanthin-Behandlung* signed with A. G. as author and written in English, it reads *"From the case histories presented, one gains the impression that many patients who have benefited subjectively from oral Strophanthin ("Strophoral") did not suffer from any cardiovascular disorder at all but more likely from various forms and degrees of psychiatric disorders"* [A.G.1951]. In 1967, Schimert published a *Klinische Symptomatologie der Herzinsuffizienz* (clinical symptomatology of heart failure), which strictly differentiates between right and left failure and is largely identical to Kern's theory of heart failure. He did not mention Kern [Schimert 1967].

Boehringer recommended Strophoral for symptons described by Kern:

- mild heart failure
- follow-up and interval treatment of severe heart insufficiencies compensated by intravenous Kombetin treatment
- stenocardic symptoms
- interval treatment of angina pectoris
- heart failure prophylaxis

In medical practice, the term *small heart therapy* was used for these indications. For the university clinicians, however, this was an indication *"which can hardly be regarded as an indication for cardiac glycosides."* [Boros 1951]. Therefore, university clinicians preferred to test Strophoral on patients with edematous heart failure. The excellent effect of intravenous Strophanthin in this indication was undisputed. In order to achieve effects in these patients with orally administered

Strophoral, doses of up to more than 30 milligrams per day had to be administered. From this it was concluded that oral Strophanthin, as described in the textbooks, is not suitable for a meaningful therapy. *"It is known that the full Digitalis dose of Strophanthin, administered intravenously, is 0.8 mg at most 1 mg. Thus, according to Kern, ten-fold quantities must be given perorally. This alone proves that the resorbability of the Strophoral, if it is taken up at all in heart-effective amounts, must be very low; it is therefore no better than that of the Strophanthin tincture"*. [Boros 1951]. A comparison of the Strophoral dosages listed by Aschenbrenner with the dosages of historical ouabain preparations does indeed prove a far-reaching conformity [Aschenbrenner 1951]. Regardless of the medical indications for which the preparations were tested, these dosage data show no advantage of Strophoral over older preparations.

Author	Single dose (mg)	Daily dose (mg)
Schedel (1904)	3.75 - 7.5	7,5 - 22,5
High home (1906)	2.5 - 5.0	30
Linzenmeier (1909)	5 - 10	30 – 40
John's son (1914)	1 - 1.5	3 – 4,5
cooper (1929)	2 - 2,5	7,5
Thiroloix (1935)	3 - 5	20
Clerc (1936)	7,5 – 10	30
Lucquin (1936)	10 - 20	30 – 40
Dimitracoff (1939)	1,2	1,2
Gigon (1940)	2 – 3	7,5
Barth (1941)	2 – 2,5	6 – 7,5
Strophoral	*3 – 6*	*20 – 30*

Therefore, no therapeutic advantages were seen in comparison to the Digitalis preparations frequently used in practice: *"Due to poor and in individual cases difficult to oversee absorption conditions, this new cardiac agent is so uncertain in comparison to intravenous Strophanthin therapy and oral treatment with Purpurea and Lanata glycosides that we do not believe it is possible to speak of a revival of oral Strophanthus therapy. ... Whether Strophoral will really prove its worth in the borderline cases of mild heart failure, in which the need for glycosides has always been a controversial issue, must be taught by the future* [Aschenbrenner 1951].

Boehringer maintained its de-escalation strategy and no longer actively participated in the Strophoral dispute. Stroporal's sales were satisfactory. Slight concessions were made with regard to perlingual application and indication. In the appendix to the documentation *"Für und Wider die orale Strophanthintherapie"* Boehringer emphasizes that "Strophoral is particularly effective in mild forms of heart failure. However, the perlingual application has not proven itself in animal experiments and in practice to such an extent that it is still to be recommended exclusively. The absorption of the Strophoral in the gastrointestinal tract is undoubtedly better than from the oral cavity." In 1954, Boehringer expanded its range of cardiac drugs with a commercially sucessful digoxin preparation, *Lanicor.* So why engage in a niche product? In 1971 a chemically modified digoxin (β-methyldigoxin) was launched. Under the trade name *Lanitop,* this product soon became one of the best-selling cardiac glycosides in Germany. The distribution of Strophoral was stopped.

Despite strong criticism from university clinicians, Strophoral has revived oral Strophanthin therapy in Germany. Other companies launched new products, some of them significantly better than Strophoral. The daily dose of Strophoral was often 20 - 30 mg ouabain [Halhuber 1954], for the Purostrophan-Dragées 2 - 6 mg per day were sufficient [Wiesend 1956]. The daily dose of Strophoperm of 1 - 2 mg was in the order of magnitude of the iv-applied Strophanthin [Altmann 1952]. In 1955 Weber published an overview of the positive clinical experiences with these preparations, which were improved over Strophoral [Weber 1955]. However, the dispute over bioavailability and suitable indications remained constant companions of orally administered Strophanthin.

The experimental determination of the bioavailability of orally administered Strophanthin still posed major difficulties in the 1950s. The detection limit of the available analytical methods was above the therapeutic concentrations. For this reason, an attempt was made to determine the resorbability of the active ingredients by determining electrocardiac changes. After oral administration of Digitalis preparations, characteristic changes can be seen in the ECG of the patients: Lowering of the ST distance and flattening of the T-wave. This "Digitalis ECG" is also observed after intravenous administration of high-dose Strophanthin. Strophoral showed no changes in the ECG even in high doses. Thus it seemed that experimental proof had been provided that no cardiac effects could be achieved with Strophoral [Reindell 1952]. However, Altmann was able to show with high-dose Strophoperm (3 - 4 mg instead of the therapeutic dose of 1 - 2 mg per day) that the characteristic ECG changes can also be forced with suitable oral Strophanthin preparations [Altmann 1952 b]. However, these changes in the ECG were accompanied by toxic symptoms (bradycardia, extrasystoles). With high doses of Purostrophan-Dragées (20 mg instead of the therapeutic 6 - 10 mg), no changes in the ST pathway or the T-wave were observed. Instead, the transition time PQ was extended and the QT duration shortened. Toxic side effects were not observed [Roth 1955]. Two decades later, Belz in 1984 [Belz 1984] and von Ardenne in 1976 [Ardenne 1976] confirmed these results with further Strophanthin preparations.

For a long time, changes in the ECG after administration of Digitalis agents were regarded as evidence of a therapeutic cardiac effect. The technical progress in diagnostic tools had Fraenkel's question *"Are we at all entitled to conclude from the toxic effect of a Digitalis body on the frog's heart on its therapeutic effect on humans?"* reformulated: *"Are we entitled to conclude from changes in the ECG on the therapeutic effect of Digitalis?"* In clinical practice, this question was unreservedly answered in the affirmative for many years. In the 1970s, it was observed that the characteristic ST changes in the ECG also occur during exercise examinations (ergometry) of healthy heart patients to whom Digitalis had been administered [Haasis 1983]. Medicines cannot have therapeutic effects on healthy people. Effects observed on healthy people are undesirable side effects. The ST changes in the ECG must therefore be interpreted as an indication of toxic side effects. The lack of Digitalis ECG after oral ouabain administration is not evidence of lack of therapeutic effects. It shows that, in contrast to oral Digitalis preparations, no toxic side effects occur with suitable ouabain preparations in therapeutic doses. The therapeutic width of ouabain is significantly greater than that of Digitalis. The fundamental problem of objectively measuring the therapeutic effect of active substances remained. The experimental determination of toxic effects of active substances had been refined by technical progress. The assessment of the therapeutic effect was reserved for subjective observation by the physician at the bedside.

Digitaloids

k-Strophanthin	Glukose – Glukose - Cymarose		k-Strophanthidin
Cymarin	Cymarose		
Convallatoxin	Rhamnose		

| Ouabain (g-Strophanthin) | Rhamnose | | g-Strophanthidin |

86

In 1961 Roland Niedner in his *"Taschenbuch der Digitalis-Therapie"* (Pocket Book of Digitalis Therapy) described the practical experiences of doctors with orally administered *Digitaloids* (Ouabain, Cymarin, Convallatoxin) [Niedner 1961]. The oral Digitaloids are completely safe to use. They are easy to dose and therefore particularly suitable for outpatient treatment. Their dosage is within wide limits without toxic symptoms as a result of overdose. The overdose symptoms known from Digitalis glycosides such as bradycardia, extrasystoles, blockages, do not occur in Digitaloids. Niedner emphasizes that blood pressure increases are often observed in Digitalis treatments. In contrast, Digitaloids often lower blood pressure. The decisive disadvantage of orally administered Digitaloids is their low absorption rate.

Bioavailability

Until well into the 1980s a high bioavailability of an active ingredient in medicine was considered a prerequisite for reliable therapeutic efficacy. The higher the percentage of active ingredient absorbed by the body, the better the effect. The bioavailability of orally administered ouabain was highly controversial and dominated the discussion about oral ouabain therapy for decades. The very low concentrations in which ouabain is already effective for a long time were below the detection limit of the available analytical methods. Although in specific cases the detection of orally applied ouabain in the blood of treated animals was qualitatively possible, quantitative data were not possible [Altmann 1952].

The bioavailability of orally administered ouabain has been repeatedly determined using constantly refined methods. In many cases, resorption in animals was determined by comparing lethal doses after intravenous and oral administration [overview in Ruiz-Torres 1970]. All these methods were subject to large uncertainties due to the indirect, differential determination of biological parameters. Only with the introduction of radioactive labelling of substances and immuno-chemical methods did direct quantitative determinations of the active substances become possible.

Using radioactively labelled substances, animal experiments have shown that ouabain and Digitalis active substances are absorbed in the small intestine. The uptake of ouabain after direct application to the tied rat intestine was 48 percent after one hour and 24 percent in the guinea pig intestine [Forth 1969]. Several studies have shown that the cardiac glycosides do not only enter the body through passive diffusion through the intestinal wall. Especially the polar (water-soluble) active ingredients are probably also actively absorbed by specific transporters.

By direct determination, very different bioavailabilities have been determined for the Strophanthus active ingredients after oral application.

Results in guinea pigs:

Garbe 1968	Ouabain 15%
Strobach 1986	Ouabain 4%, k-Strophanthin 16%
Leuschner 2001	Ouabain 43 – 50%

Results in humans:

Marchetti 1971	Ouabain 10 %
Ghirardi 1973	k-Strophanthin 22% after 5h, 31% after 24 h
Greeff 1974	Ouabain 2%
Erdle 1979	Ouabain 1.2 – 5%

Regardless of differences in the details of measurement methods (time of measurement, applied dose) and the use of different Strophanthin preparations, these results leave no doubt that Strophanthus drugs, especially ouabain, have low inherent bioavailabilities.

Berthold Kern had hoped that the detection of sufficiently high absorption of oral Strophanthin would increase the acceptance of his theory of heart failure. He therefore personally took part in some measurements. Gross, University of Heidelberg, and his doctoral student Erdle investigated the resorption of radioactively labelled ouabain. Kern was personally present at the measurements, as he wrote in a letter of March 18, 1978: *"In the second attempt on humans I was present myself: the Strodival paste, 99.9 mg with 6% ouabain was applied to the dried tongue, after about 1 minute during which the mouth remained open, the mouth was closed and the paste still present was distributed throughout the mouth with the usual tongue movement, exactly in the type of therapeutic application. ... As far as the measurement of the first human experiment already allows a statement, urine excretion seems to be around 1%"*. The results of the Erdle study were devastating for Kern: less than 5% absorption after oral administration of ouabain! [Erdle 1979].

Despite the clear results, Kern remained convinced that orally administered ouabain is absorbed 100 percent by the body. He saw himself strengthened in this view by a test which he already had carried out at the Württembergisches Landesuntersuchungsamt in 1952. A color test in the intestines of test persons who had received orally administered Strophoral had not been able to detect any ouabain. Kern concluded from this test that the Strophoral administered had been completely absorbed [Kern 1952]. He therefore demanded that with the new analysis methods, not only the active substance absorbed by the body but also the fate of the part not absorbed should be determined. Such measurements have not been carried out. Contrary to all clear analytical results, Kern never gave up his conviction that ouabain administered orally is completely absorbed. However, his hypothesis of complete absorption was in clear contradiction to the fact that ouabain was fatal in intravenous administration at doses of 1 - 2 mg, but was easily tolerated in oral administration of 30 mg Strophoral. Kern had no plausible explanation for this contradiction. His insistence on complete absorption of oral ouabain has further deepened the gap between him and university clinicians.

Berthold Kern had always stressed in his books that scientific progress in medicine can only result from critical observation of nature and inductive thinking. He had made it his personal maxim to summarize the details of general laws from which new insights can be logically derived, observed without prejudice. To the detriment of his theory of heart failure and the subsequent pathogenesis of myocardial infarction with regard to the bioavailability of orally administered ouabain, he did not live up to this claim. Here he has fallen back to dogmatic deductive thinking: the dogma is above the facts.

Kern knew from his clinical experience that oral ouabain has an effect on humans. Despite the apparently low bioavailability of ouabain, many other clinicians had also achieved very good clinical success with orally administered ouabain preparations. Two preparations proved to be particularly effective in medical practice: the Purostrophan dragées from Kali-Chemie and the Strophoperm solution from Permicutan KG.

In early 1953, Kali-Chemie offered the dragées developed in cooperation with Mutschler, which were coated with an enteric lacquer. The dragées only dissolved in the small intestine and released the active ingredient there. With this preparation, the therapeutic dose could be greatly reduced compared to the strophoral tablets already dissolving in the stomach [Mutschler 1952]. Just one year later, Kali-Chemie improved Purostrophan again. A substance (sodium-laurylsulphate) was added to the dragées to reduce the surface tension of water. This increased the solubility of ouabain in water by a factor of four and the dissolution rate by a factor of 7.5. In tests on dogs, it was shown that the time to onset of effect after application of the dragées was significantly shortened. The individual scattering of the measurement results was significantly smaller than that of the dragées without sodium-laurylsulfate [Krause 1955]. These observations have also been confirmed many times in therapeutic applications.

The addition of synthetic sodium-laurylsulfate was modelled on reports on the improvement of the effects of Strophanthus preparations by adding natural surface-active substances. As early as 1925 it had been reported that the addition of saponins improved the resorption of Strophanthin in the small intestine [Wiesend 1956-b]. Like sodium-laurylsulfate, saponins are surface-active substances (surfactants). One part of the saponin molecule is water-soluble, another is fat-soluble. Due to this chemical structure, they reduce the surface tension of the water in a similar way to soap. *(Sapo* is the Latin word for soap). Saponins usually taste bitter and cause irritation of the mucous membrane. They are widespread in the plant world. They are abundant in many plants used as food. Digitonin, a saponin commonly used for research purposes, is found in the Red Foxglove seed along with Digitalis glycosides. The seeds of Strophathus plants also contain saponins. Saponins have a special property: they increase the permeability of cell membranes. This property is the reason for the improvement of the absorbability of Strophanthin in the small intestine after the addition of saponins. Fraser had therefore had good experiences with the Strophanthus tincture. This also explains why Fraenkel and other physicians have reported better effects of Strophanthus tincture compared to pure active ingredients. The variable effect of the tincture was due to the preparation, which, as it was not standardized, contained saponins that promoted absorption, sometimes more and sometimes less. However, the saponins also contributed to the incompatibility and the known severe side effects of the tincture due to irritation of the mucous membranes. In the 1970s Herbert GmbH launched ouabain preparations under the trade name *Strodival*. These preparations contained lecitine (phospholipids) as surface-active substances. Phospholipids are present in every cell of the human body. They form the main component of the cell membrane and also have a variety of biological functions.

Compared to all other ouabain preparations, the *Strophoperm* of Permicutan KG allowed by far the lowest dose. Dosages of 1 - 2 mg per day were sufficient in most cases for an effect comparable to that of intravenous administration [Altmann 1952, Kotsovsky1953, Burger 1953]. The exact composition of the Strophoperm solution is not known. Permicutan only revealed general information on the composition in a Strophoperm brochure: *"Strophoperm contains 4 mg in 1 cc solution, i.e. 0.4 mg in the average dose of 3 drops. The solvent takes into account the physical conditions and physiological processes of perlingual absorption of active substances. A good penetration into the surface is achieved by increased wetting capability, by the body's own electrolytes, with which the cell controls the permeability of its interface, favourable osmotic conditions are achieved and by suitable buffering a stabilization to the required pH value. The necessary Strophanin doses in Strophoperm are only slightly above the i. v. applied amounts, which can only be explained by an optimal, rapid absorption"*. Reference is made to measurements by A. Sjoerdsma, University of Chicago, which he presented at a pharmacological congress in Gothenburg in 1955. In his tests, radioactively labelled ouabain is absorbed to 45 percent from Strophoperm solution within 60 minutes. The Sjoerdsma lecture has apparently not been published in writing. The data are supported by Maehder, who measured the absorption of radioactively labelled Strophanthidin acetate (the sugar chain on the aglycone of ouabain is replaced by an acetic acid residue) from Strophoperm solvent in guinea pigs in 1955. He reports a resorption of 55 percent [Maehder 1955].

These experiences with the various ouabain preparations all confirmed the observation described by Berthold Kern in 1951 that *"the same glycoside in the same dosage and application to the same person can have a strong effect, depending on the nature of the vehicle indifferent per se, but can also have little or no effect"*. [Kern 1951, p. 17]. The preparations all contained the same active ingredient, ouabain, they differed only in the *indifferent vehicles*. Berthold Kern was personally present at the Erdle tests in Heidelberg. There he was able to observe that the absorption of ouabain from alcoholic solution was different from that from Strodival paste. In a letter dated May 27, 1978, he asked the right question: *"Why do they differ so much depending on the carrier material?"* But instead of exploring the function of the indifferent vehicle, which he had recognized to be important as early as 1951, he repeatedly falls for the error of a rather unhelpful rejection of measuring methods. From today's perspective, it is no longer understandable why, despite the clear experimental and clinical experience, the importance of additives for bioavailability has not been considered in the discussion about oral ouabain therapy by critics and supporters. The dogma of a high bioavailability of active substances as a prerequisite for reliable therapeutic efficacy had apparently become firmly anchored in the minds of physicians.

~ ~ ~

The years 1960 to 1990 were the *golden age* for Digitalis glycosides. They were not only the standard medication for heart failure, they were among the most frequently prescribed drugs worldwide. Many companies launched digoxin and digitoxin based products. Although they all contained the same amount of active ingredient per tablet, poisoning often occurred when switching from one product to another. In 1971, Lindenbaum and his team were able to show that not only digoxin preparations from different suppliers had different efficacy qualities. Even different batches from the same manufacturer showed clear differences [Lindenbaum 1971]. Even minor changes in the composition of the tablets led to significant differences in effect.

Subsequently, tests carried out on preparations on the market revealed drastic differences in serum concentrations. Patients who were adjusted to preparations with low potency suffered digoxin poisoning after switching to preparations with higher potency.

Serum digoxin levels after oral application of various digoxin preparations

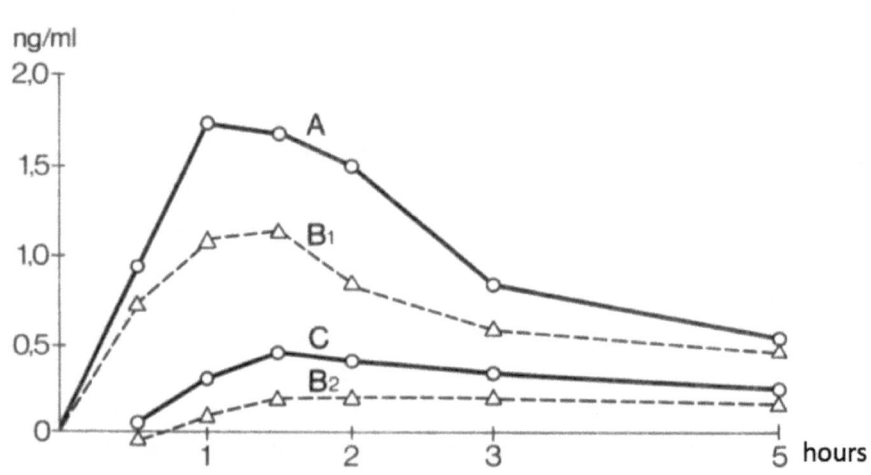

Digoxin tablets from various manufacturers (A and C)
and 2 batches from the same manufacturer (B^1 and B^2]

These observations brought the importance of galenics for the quality of drug action into the interest of pharmaceutical companies and regulatory authorities. Dramatic differences in release and absorption depending on the formulation had also been found for other active ingredients. In order to guarantee the interchangeability of preparations with identical active substances, *bioequivalence* must be demonstrated for new preparations with the same active substance in Germany since 1988. Medicinal products are bioequivalent if the extent and rate of drug absorption are comparable. Only then can it be assumed that an exchange between the drugs can take place without endangering the patient. Bioequivalence is of great importance for generics, the products offered by companies after the expiration of patents for original preparations, often at drastically lower prices. Today, the optimization of the dosage forms of active ingredients through suitable additives is an essential part of the development of a drug. Extensive tests of pharmaceutical quality must be carried out and the quality of the preparations must be proven in the approval procedure.

Cardiac glycoside tablets contain less than one milligram of active ingredient per tablet. With a total weight of 100 mg they consist of more than 99% indifferent excipients. With these, properties such as resorbability can be optimized. Important for this are dissolution rate and solubility, which can be influenced by various parameters: crystalline or amorphous state of the active substance, particle size, integration into a solvent matrix, etc. In addition, the mechanical stability and shelf life of the tablet must be guaranteed. In addition to fillers, a tablet contains binders, flow regulators, lubricants, hydrophilising and disintegrating agents. The latter are agents that cause the tablet to disintegrate rapidly after contact with water. All of these aids, known as *galenics,* offer the possibility of optimizing the bioavailability of active ingredients.

According to current knowledge, the absolute bioavailability of an active ingredient is not an essential condition for a good therapeutic effect. The bioinformatics company *PharmaInformatic* has developed a database containing all bioavailability data published worldwide for drugs. The average oral bioavailability of drugs is approx. 54 percent. In about 28 percent of medicines, it is less than 30 percent. 12 percent of all drugs have a bioavailability of less than 10 percent. These values put the importance of the absolute bioavailability of a preparation into perspective. It is of minor importance for the assessment of the systemic availability of an active substance. The only decisive question is whether serum concentrations can be achieved with a galenic dosage form after oral administration which are necessary for a therapeutic effect and can be maintained for a longer period of time. In many cases, even small absolute bioavailabilities are sufficient for this.

Many top-selling drugs have only moderate absolute bioavailability. The antihypertensive Aliskiren, which was only approved a few years ago, has a bioavailability of 2.5 percent, the Dabigatran Etexilate (anticoagulant), which is still young, reaches 6.5 percent and the calcium antagonist Nisoledipine 5 percent. Even the classic ACE inhibitor Ramipril has a modest bioavailability of only 15 percent.

To ensure safe therapeutic efficacy, an active ingredient must reach a concentration in the blood above the No-Effect Level (NOEL) and below the Maximum Tolerable Dose (MTD). A high absolute bioavailability increases the probability that systemic concentrations above the NOEL can be achieved. However, it is only of primary economic importance. The higher the absolute bioavailability, the lower the required amount of active ingredient. Small amounts of active ingredient increase the profit per dose.

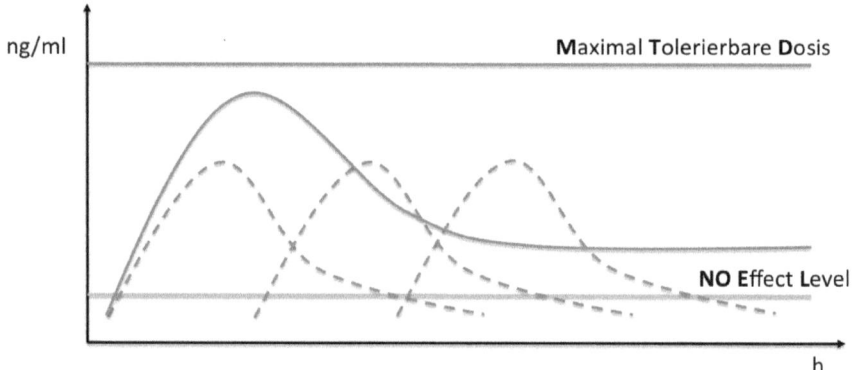

In 1990, the head of development at Herberts GmbH, Dr. Herrmann, pointed out in an article on the efficacy of oral ouabain therapy that *"pharmacologists are also concerned as to whether the assumption of a linear quantitative relationship between the calculated absorption rate and the qualitative pharmacodynamic effect of a pharmacon is permissible. Rather, they are increasingly of the opinion that it is not the systemic bioavailability that should be a criterion for pharmaceutical efficacy, but the proportion of the drug that reaches the local bio-phase."* [Herrmann 1990]. By the time this was generally recognized in medicine, it was already too late for ouabain.

~ ~ ~

Due to the resistance of university clinicians ouabain remained a niche product in post-war Germany. It was the domain of small and medium-sized enterprises. Outside Germany, oral ouabain preparations were hardly used any more. The major research-based pharmaceutical companies concentrated on the active ingredients of Digitalis. Attempts were made to find more effective and, above all, less toxic derivatives by modifying the chemical structure. No fundamental changes in the structure have been successful. Small changes in the sugar chains of digoxin - methylation and acetylation - made it possible to produce active ingredients that were easier to dose than digoxin itself. These products included Novodigal (β-acetyl-digoxin), Sandolanide (α-acetyl-digoxin) and Lanitop (β-methyl-digoxin). These preparations have in common that they are immediately cleaved after absorption in the body and release digoxin. Novodigal and Lanitop were by far the most frequently prescribed drugs in Germany in 1982. Strophanthin preparations were not included in the list of the 500 most frequently prescribed drugs. Germany was the stronghold of the Digitalis prescriptions. In 1977, 60 times more Digitalis preparations were prescribed in Germany than in the USA and 80 times more than in England in relation to the total population. Poisoning symptoms occurred in about 20 percent of the patients treated.

Myocardial Infarction

Heart attack - like hardly any other term, this word is associated with fear, terror and death. Almost 300,000 people suffer a heart attack in Germany every year. About 65,000 of them are fatal. The term heart attack (or myocardial infarction) refers to diseases of the heart that lead to the death of heart muscle cells. When large areas of the heart muscle die, the heart stops functioning and the patient dies. If the death of heart muscle cells is restricted to smaller areas, the patient survives the heart attack. According to the current textbook presentation, a heart attack is the result of a persistent circulatory disorder of the heart. It is caused by arteriosclerosis of the coronary vessels, the arteries that supply the heart muscle with blood (coronary arteries). Arteriosclerosis is the term used to describe deposits of blood fats and cholesterol in the arterial walls. These cause stiffening of the vessel walls and result in a reduction of the arterial diameter. The blood circulation in the heart muscle is disturbed. The supply of the heart with oxygen and nutrients is no longer sufficiently guaranteed. When the sclerotic deposits in the artery walls (plaques) tear, the body activates blood clotting. Blood clots form which completely seal off the already narrowed coronary arteries. The blood circulation stops. The heart cells die. In many cases of heart attacks, however, no blood clots (thromboses) can be detected.

Heart attack is a modern phenomenon. The frequency of heart attacks has increased a hundredfold in the 20th century. Before the Second World War, heart attack was nothing more than a side note even in textbooks. In 1946, Berthold Kern also dedicated only a few lines to heart attacks in his book *Grundlagen der Inneren Medizin*. He describes it as a *particularly severe angina pectoris attack caused by arteriosclerosis of the large and medium coronary artery strains*. For therapy he referred to cardiac glycosides, namely Strophanthin, which were often beneficial. It was assumed that they promote coronary blood flow.

The first prominent heart attack patient in medical history, of whom there is an exact medical history and an autopsy report, must have been John Hunter, anatomist and surgeon at St. Georg Hospital in London [Aschenbrenner 1956]. He is described as a *restless worker*. He had suffered from angina pectoris since he was 48 years old. In 1793, at the age of 65, he died suddenly in the morning in his hospital after an annoying confrontation. In the autopsy report it is noted: *"the pericardium was found to be unnaturally thickened... 2 matt white spots in the aortic chamber, 1.5 inches in square, ... the wreath arteries at the outlet ossified."* Two of the observations mentioned in the Hunter case still determine the discussion about the causes of heart attacks:

annoying confrontation = emotional excitement, stress and

Wreath arteries ossified = coronary occlusion, which prevents the oxygen supply to the heart.

These observations lead to two different interpretations of the development of heart attacks. The *myocardial model* (myocardial theory) sees the cause of the heart attack in diseases of the heart muscle. The *coronary model* (coronary theory) suspects the cause of the heart attack in a circulatory disorder of the heart muscle. It is known that stress and emotional excitation can damage the heart muscle by releasing high doses of stress hormones. John Hunter suffered his heart attack after an angry quarrel, so he was under stress. This finding is important in the myocardial model. Corpse dissection revealed calcifications of the coronary arteries. This finding is important in the coronary model. The discussion about the *correct* causes of a heart attack, whether coronary or myocardial, has been very doggedly debated in medicine.

It was only after the Second World War that doctors became aware of the threatening extent of heart attacks. In many hospitals, the number of patients with heart attacks multiplied in the 1950s compared to the numbers before the war. Aschenbrenner writes in 1956:

> "In the last 10 years, the question of optimal heart attack treatment has come to the forefront of medical and public interest in many countries of the world ("manager's disease"). There can be no doubt that myocardial infarction in its classic form has not only been diagnosed more frequently since the late 1930s, but that it has actually increased in frequency in many countries with a high standard of living. Rushing and pressing responsibility, constant overload with sleep deficit, renouncement of sufficient vacation, nicotine and coffee abuse certainly play an important role in the complex causal structure of the myocardial infarction. These sociological influences of the technical century were already clearly recognized by William Osler in 1910. He spoke - even then! - from the "high pressure life" in the times of modern ocean steamships (Lusitania!) and also attributed angina pectoris as a medicorum disease to the "treadmill" of the medical practice". [Aschenbrenner 1956].

Heart attacks also became increasingly important in medical research after the Second World War. Causes and therapy options were sought. As Aschenbrenner put it, post-war living conditions, characterized by stress-inducing conditions, were initially regarded as the main cause of the dramatic increase in heart attacks. In addition, arteriosclerosis soon became the focus of interest.

The activities of the heart are controlled by the autonomic nervous system. The sympathetic nervous system acts as a mediator between environment and circulation. It translates external stimuli into internal stimulation of the cardiovascular system. Catecholamines - epinephrine, norepinephrine - are the messenger substances that transmit the neuronal impulses of the sympathetic nervous system on a molecular level. Heart damaging effects of catecholamines were discovered very early on. As early as 1905, several research groups had shown that epinephrine induced heart muscle necrosis (death of heart muscle cells) in animal experiments. Wilhelm Raab (1895 - 1970), University of Vermont, in 1927 had made a self-experiment *("because rabbits or even dogs were too expensive"!)*. Subcutaneous injection of 1.3 mg epinephrine had triggered an *"excessively painful, typical angina pectoris attack with severe acute ECG changes and subsequent collapse"* [Raab 1966]. Hans Selye (1907-1982), founder of stress research, proved in the 1950s with a series of fundamental studies that subliminal catecholamine doses, as well as catecholamine releases caused by stress, in combination with mineralocorticoids cause severe necrosis in the heart muscle [Selye 1961]. In animal experiments, heart muscle necrosis could be triggered in rats with emotional stress [Raab 1964]. After exposure to high epinephrine doses, lactate[6] was paradoxically found in coronary sinus blood despite high oxygen saturation as it is also observed in coronary sinus blood of angina pectoris patients [Bretschneider 1956]. Gremels had already described the stimulating effect of catecholamines on heart metabolism in the 1930s.

Epinephrine is produced in the adrenal gland. Radiation of the adrenal gland with X-rays can reduce the release of epinephrine in the adrenal gland. With this method Raab achieved good results in the treatment of angina pectoris patients [Raab 1950]. From these findings and similar results of other researchers it was concluded that ischemic conditions of the heart muscle (angina pectoris, coronary heart disease, heart attack) are not caused solely by disturbances of the arterial oxygen supply to the heart muscle. The influence of increased catecholamines released under stress on the degree of myocardial oxygen consumption must also be taken into account.

An increased oxygen consumption of the heart muscle caused by catecholamine release is usually compensated by an expansion of the coronary arteries, which promotes blood circulation. The stretching of the arteries allows an increased blood and oxygen supply and thus

---

[6] Lactate is often interpreted in medicine as an indication of oxygen deficiency.

compensates for the increased consumption. Only when this protective reflex is no longer guaranteed by a stiffening of the arteries, the metabolism of the heart muscle derails. The more the coronary arteries' elasticity is restricted by arteriosclerosis, the more dangerous are too high catecholamine concentrations. Circulatory disorders of the heart caused by arteriosclerosis are therefore not the trigger for the metabolic processes leading to a heart attack; they are merely a risk factor. People with arteriosclerosis of the heart arteries have a higher risk of heart attack than people without arteriosclerosis.

On the basis of these findings, Raab formulated in 1966 that for many scientists the pathogenesis of heart attacks had actually been clarified:

> "Today, however, things stand in such a way that despite many still ongoing ambiguities in detail, the traditional, one-sided mechanistic notions of a purely vascular and haemo-dynamically caused development of "coronary" ischemic and degenerative heart diseases have been abandoned by many leading researchers in favor of a "pluricausal" concept that emphasizes the metabolism." [Raab 1966][7].

However, this conclusion was not shared by all researchers. Epidemiological surveys in the USA in the 1950s indicated a link between fatty diets and the incidence of cardiovascular disease. It has been postulated that high-fat food increases the risk of heart disease. In particular, a high cholesterol diet (meat, eggs, milk, butter and other dairy products) leads to an increased cholesterol level. The elevated cholesterol level in turn causes arteriosclerosis and thus through circulatory disorders heart failure and heart attack. This line of argument met with a particularly positive response in the USA.

---

[7] Raab published a detailed description of the effects of catecholamines on the heart in 1963: Raaab W, The nonvascular metabolic myocardial vulnerability factor in "coronary heart disease". Fundamentals of pathogenesis, treatment and prevention Am Heart J. 1963; 66: 685-706.

The historian Peter Stearns pointed out that a *diet culture* was already firmly anchored in America at the beginning of the twentieth century. Especially for white women of the middle and upper middle classes, slim bodies were the preferred ideal of beauty. Calorie counting was the preferred approach to do this justice. The postulate of a connection between a high-fat diet and heart disease promoted the acceptance of low-fat diets. Science organizations and government agencies fuelled this trend.

Although the fat and cholesterol hypothesis was scientifically controversial, in 1957 the American Heart Association issued a recommendation to limit the consumption of fatty products in order to reduce the risk of coronary heart disease. The recommendation restrictively emphasised that *"there is still no definitive evidence that heart attacks or strokes can be prevented by these measures"*. But the controversial hypothesis did take on a life of its own in the scientific debate. It was soon considered proven. In the official US Dietary Guidelines of the US government, which are updated every five years, high-fat and cholesterol foods were classified as a risk for cardiovascular diseases.

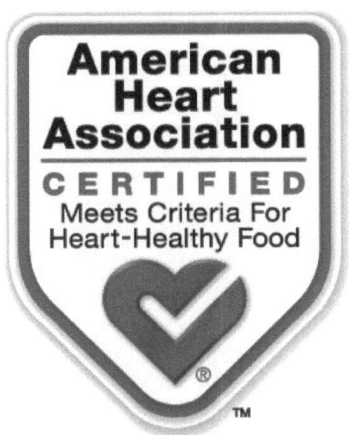

Certificate of the American Heart Association for healthy food

In 1961, the American Heart Association included a warning of cholesterol in its guidelines. In 1977, cholesterol was officially classified as a potentially harmful component of food in the US Department of Health's Dietary Goals, which should be minimized. In 1985, several research organizations initiated a National Cholesterol Education Program (NCEP). An upper limit of 300 milligrams of cholesterol per day (about two eggs) has been set in the USA and Switzerland. If you eat more, you dig your own grave.

With reference to scientific findings, the food industry promoted fat and cholesterol-reduced products for the prevention of heart diseases. The

American Heart Association certified suitable foods that could be advertised with a special logo. Low-fat nutrition has become an ideology.

With her book *The Big Fat Surprise: Why Butter, Meat and Cheese Belong in a Healthy Diet,* Nina Teicholz has written a very readable popular-scientific presentation of the origin of the fat and cholesterol myth [Teicholz 2015]. It shows how speculative scientific hypotheses have been transformed into a dogmatic worldview. Based on dubious statistical evaluations of epidemiological studies, political actionism led to a combination of health care and the economic interests of the food industry. Ulrike Gonder and Nicolay Worm prove in their book *Mehr Fett: Liebeserklärung an einen verteufelten Nährstoff* (More fat: declaration of love to a devilish nutrient) that in Germany as well manipulative interpretations of epidemiological studies have led to proliferation of the fat and cholesterol myths. [Gonder 2010].

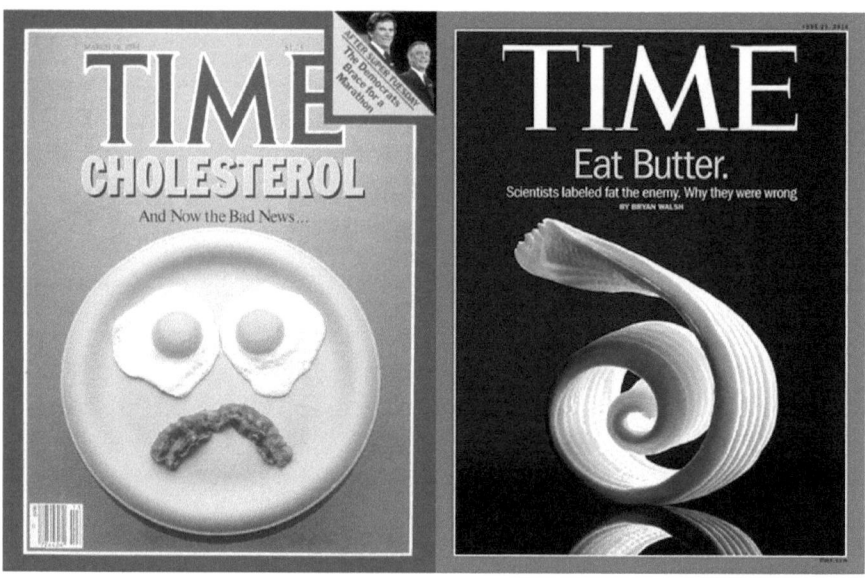

Title page TIME, March 26, 1984
Cholesterol and fat are bad

Title page TIME, June 23, 2014
Fat-rich food is good

Currently there are signs of a reversal. In 2008, the UN Food and Agriculture Organization and the World Health Organization, WHO, in a joint evaluation of all available studies, concluded: *"that there is no probable or convincing evidence of significant effects of dietary fats on coronary heart disease or cancer."* [WHO 2008]. The draft of the US Dietary Guidelines 2015 states that there is no evidence of a connection between diet and cholesterol in blood levels. Cholesterol is no longer considered a questionable component of food. The 6th Swiss Nutrition Report from 2012 also gave an all-clear signal *"From a scientific point of view, no concrete restriction of cholesterol intake in mg/day can be recommended"*. The consumption of cholesterol-containing foods such as eggs, butter or cheese does not increase the cholesterol level in the blood.

The cholesterol hypothesis was supported by findings in patients who had died of heart attack. Clogged arteries (thrombosis) could be detected in a high percentage of cases. This consolidated the still valid doctrine that an acute occlusion of a heart artery by a blood clot triggers the heart attack.

The main focus of the fat and cholesterol hypothesis was supply of oxygen to the heart muscle. The consumption of oxygen was (and is) masked out. No one will attempt to evaluate the financial situation of a person or company by exclusively considering revenue and neglecting expenditure. However, this error of thought has dominated the discussion about the pathogenesis of *coronary* heart diseases for decades. Only the income - blood circulation - is evaluated. Expenditure - oxygen consumption - is not considered. The oxygen consumption must not be equated with the oxygen demand. Supply and demand are independent of the ability of the heart muscle to utilize oxygen. A disturbance of the heart's ability to utilize oxygen cannot be compensated by an increased supply of oxygen. No matter how high the supply and demand, a deficit cannot be compensated if the heart cannot process oxygen.

In Germany, the influential Heidelberg internist Gotthard Schettler was particularly committed to the cholesterol hypothesis. In an interview with DER SPIEGEL on October 28, 1964 he stated:

"There has always been a heart attack, but in recent decades the rate of infarct death in all so-called civilized countries has increased rapidly and sharply, including the Soviet Union, Poland and Hungary. And today we know for sure: A large part of cardiovascular diseases is favoured, initiated and maintained by disorders of the fat balance in the body."

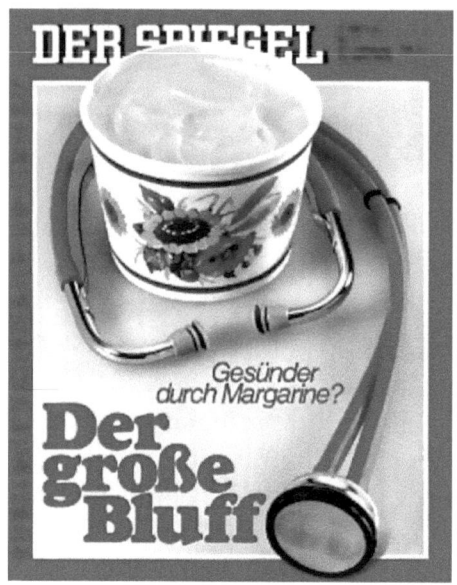

Cover of DER SPIEGEL
April 23, 1979

Schettler maintained close relations with the margarine industry. The "Margarine-Institut für gesunde Ernährung" distributed reprints of Schettler publications to doctors, journalists and other multitiplicators as background information on the positive effects of unsaturated fatty acids. Following recommendations by Schettler, the Margarine Institute awarded the "Heinrich-Wieland-Prize" worth 15,000 marks each year. In 1989, Schettler himself was awarded the Heinrich Wieland Prize for his life's work. With a controversial paper entitled *"Risk factors, dietary fats and degenerative cardiovascular diseases"*, Schettler initially succeeded in involving the German Medical Association in his efforts for the margarine industry. When the German Research Foundation distanced itself from this Schettler paper because *"it cannot be excluded"* that *"commercial interests in individual cases have led to a one-sided presentation of scientific results or even to the dissemination of unproven assumptions"*, the German Medical Association distanced itself from Schettler and his colleagues. Prof. Edmund Renner from Giessen formulated his criticism even more clearly. He described the margarine advocates among his medical colleagues simply as "corruptible".

On April 29, 1996 the SPIEGEL wrote in an obituary for Schettler:

> "For over 20 years, from 1963 to 1986, the Heidelberg internist was the most influential German doctor. He made cholesterol a villain in the heart-attack drama and at the same time offered the frightened citizens a therapy: margarine instead of butter. Although the scientific evidence was extremely poor, Schettler succeeded in persuading the majority of his peers of his class to accept the thesis of the blessing of polyunsaturated fatty acids. ... Schettler's Heidelberg "Internist School" resulted in a dozen full professorships and more than 100 senior physicians."

Schettler and his students played a decisive role in establishing the doctrine in Germany that an acute occlusion of a heart artery damaged by arteriosclerosis triggers heart attack.

Berthold Kern and Left Myocardiology

In his theory of heart failure Berthold Kern in 1948 had referred to the special position of the left ventricles in the development of heart failure. In the 1960s he expanded the theory of left heart failure to a more comprehensive *left myocardiology*. In 1968 his book *Der Myokardinfarkt* (Myocardial Infarction) was published. Therein Kern discusses the development of myocardial infarction and its prevention through timely oral ouabain therapy [Kern 1974]. He formulated his findings briefly and concisely in the preamble to the book

> "Coronary theory is dead. The fact that myocardial infarction is not caused by coronary anomalies is proven, even statistically proven, by the overwhelming abundance of medical research results from three human generations.
>
> Myocardial theory has replaced it. The fact that left ventricular myocardial infarction always arises from myocardial anomalies of the left ventricle has been completely clarified by an astonishing wealth of university medical research results on left myocardiology in recent decades.
>
> Again and again consequent thinking yielded mercilessly: who knows, recognizes and acknowledges even fractions of the supposedly new left mycardiology, there is scientifically no return to the old familiar coronary theory, to coronary heart disease.
>
> So all that remains is a worldwide reversal. This conversion, the revocation of the coronary doctrine from our own earlier books has also been difficult for us. But when serving the sick, the truth leaves no other choice."

Kern leaves no doubt that he is concerned with the correct knowledge, the truth, which results from observing nature, logic and consistent thinking. He regards doubts about his left myocardiology as absurd because *they run counter to natural conditions.*

The starting point of Kern's left myocardiology is the specificity of the heart attack to the left ventricle. A heart attack almost always starts in the left ventricle. Therefore, similar to heart failure, Kern strictly differentiates between infarcts of the right and left ventricle. The left ventricle contracts in the systole and thereby presses the blood into the circulation. The inner layers of the left ventricle are inevitably "white-pressed" without blood, similar to the palms of the hands during a strong fist closure. This results in a systolic blood circulation stop for the muscle cells of the left inner layers. About half of the time the inner layers are bloodless, their capillaries are compressed, all diffusion processes of oxygen, nutrients and metabolic products are prevented. Exchange of substances between the bloodstream and cells is not possible in the systole. In contrast, blood circulation is always ensured without interruption in all other sections of the heart. The systolic circulatory stop in the left inner layers is not a circulatory disorder. It is not caused by pathological changes in the cardiac arteries. It is a natural reduced blood flow caused by the functioning of the heart muscle. Kern describes this as a *time-dependent limitation of supply availability*: *"No matter how great the demand of the cell, no matter how large the supply of blood in the veins is, the less the need is satisfied, the more hindering the usability of what is offered is subject to time-dependent restrictions"*. The cells only have a small time window to absorb nutrients and release metabolic products. Even small metabolic disorders can have devastating consequences. Kern clarifies this interrelationship with the parable of the domestic water pipe:

> "A residential house represents the myocardial cell; the main pipe of the municipal water supply, which runs in the street along the house, corresponds to the supply capillary, which runs along the myocardial cell; and the supply pipe of the house brings water into the house from the supply in the street pipe by means of flow transport (analogous to diffusion trans-

port) through the house wall (cell membrane) depending on household requirements. The street pipe has a capacity of 1 m^3/min, which is sufficient for the maximum demand of the house of 0.1 m^3/min. Suddenly there is an increased demand, for example due to a fire blaze (stress with catecholamine-induced metabolic excess of many times the upper standard limit), which requires, for example, 10 m^3/min of extinguishing water. However, the pipe through the house wall (cell membrane) does not allow this much to pass inside, the house is incinerated (the cell is necrotic). The accident could also not be averted by expanding the road pipe to 200 m^3/min supply capacity (coronary dilatation) or by passing more water through the road with an additional parallel pipe (collaterals) or by connecting the pipe of this road to the pipe of a neigh-bouring road by cross-connection (anastomosis). The fire bri-gade can use additional pipes (hoses) through the house wall (doors, windows) to channel any amount of water into the house and extinguish the fire. However, more mass exchange can never pass through the cell membrane than its structure per unit of time allows. It is precisely through such "limping" that the parable of the house so clearly shows the limits of na-ture, but also the aberration of any research that runs counter to such natural conditions."

Kern consistently excludes any influence of circulatory disorders and improvements on heart attacks. Neither mechanical, stents and bypass surgery, nor drug improvements in blood flow through vasodilators such as nitro sprays, nor endogenous blood flow-promoting collate-rals[8] and anastomoses are relevant for the pathogenesis of myocardial infarction. The heart attack is triggered solely by disorders of the myocardial metabolism. The cells in the inner layer of the left ventri-

---

[8] Collaterals are a side branches in the bloodstream. They ensure the blood supply to a tissue area in the event of blockage or injury to individual blood vessels. They are connected to each other via anastomoses, so that they are often referred to as a collateral network. In addition to the coronary arteries, blood circulation in the heart is also ensured by a distinctive network of collaterals and anastomoses.

cle are particularly susceptible to failure due to their physiological function. Kern lists a number of triggering factors that can disturb the metabolism of heart cells:

- somatic stress (acute overexertion)

- mental stress (damages mainly through acute tonus increase of the sympathetic nervous system)

- acute increase of the sympathetic nervous system (stress, pain, nicotine)

- acute blood pressure crises in hypertensive patients

- tachycardia of any kind and cause (stress)

- acute myocardial damaging neural impulses from the vegetative nervous system

- acute intercurrent infections

- iatrogenic damage (Digitalis infarcts)

- combination forms

In the interpretation of Kern this pluricausal diversity of noxae acts in the myocardial cell via relatively few pathogenetic intermediate mechanisms, which lead to a uniform central disorder and weaken and cancel out the viability of the cell. Just as a conflagration can be caused by lightning, arson, short circuit and other multi-causal causes, but then carries out its work of destruction in the same way.

Kern derived his left myocardiology from a precise analysis of the heart activity and the specific requirements to which the individual heart chambers are exposed. He did not conduct any experimental studies of his own to confirm his hypotheses. Instead, he has relied on the compatibility of clinical observations and research results with his conclusions.

Theses and research on coronary theory occupy a large part of Kern's thinking. He very clearly shows the obvious contradictions of the coronary theory to many experimental and clinical findings. For his conclusion that only left myocardiology can explain the pathogenesis of myocardial infarction, however, he does not present reliable reasons. From the doubts about coronary theory it logically does not follow that only left myocardiology is correct.

Kern's central criticism of the coronary theory were experimental findings on the circulation of the heart, which were not compatible with a circulatory disorder as the trigger for the heart attack. Thrombi cannot be detected in a large number of deceased patients. Several research groups had also published findings that the longer patients lived after a heart attack, the more frequently thrombi (blood clots) occur in infarct-dead. These observations suggest that arterial occlusions caused by blood clots can[9] be the result and not the cause of heart attacks.

The research of Giorgio Baroldi played a major role in the criticism of coronary theory. Baroldi (1925 - 2007) was an award-winning Italian pathologist. After graduating in 1949 and teaching at the University of Milano (until 1959), he worked at the Armed Forces Institute of Pathology in Washington from 1960 to 1968. He then returned to Italy, where he held chairs at the universities of Pisa and Milano.

Baroldi has gained fundamental insights into the circulation of the heart. Using a special preparation technique, he was able to visualize the collateral circulation of the heart muscle. He filled the coronary arteries of deceased with a liquid plastic that cures to a solid mass when heated. The muscle flesh then was detached by an acid bath. The vascular effusions produced in this way show a variety of collaterals and anastomoses which, in addition to the coronary arteries, contribute to blood circulation in the heart muscle. Baroldi has been able

---

[9] In later studies it has been observed that the earlier the measurements are taken, the more frequently thrombi can be detected in patients who survive the heart attack. Apparently the thrombi can dissolve again (thrombolysis) which prevents a fatal heart attack. DeWood MA, Spores J, Notske R et al. Prevalence of total coronary occlusion during the early hours of transmural myocardial infarction. N Engl J Med 1980; 303: 897-902

to show that even total occlusions of a cardiac artery do not have to lead to a stopp in blood circulation. Collaterals and anastomoses assume the blood supply.

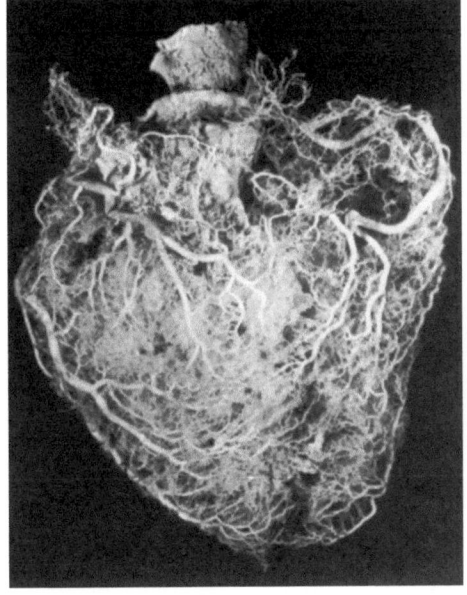 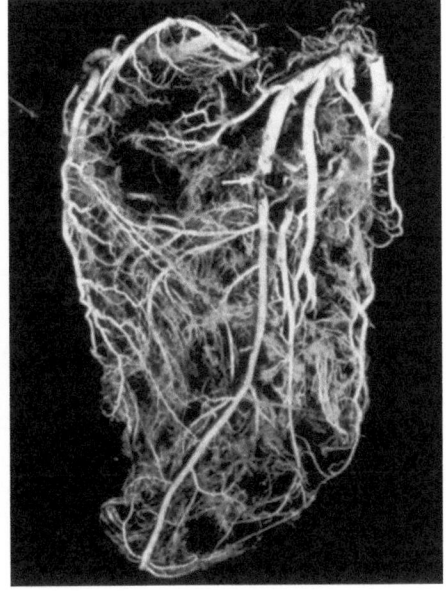

Collateral and anastomosis network of a healthy heart

total occlusion of an artery (arrow) is compensated by collaterals and anastomoses

The collateral network is a phenomenon that has been intensively researched. Patients with a well-developed collateral circulation have a lower risk of suffering a heart attack than patients with a less well-developed [Seiler 2014]. However, the collateral circulation cannot compensate for an acute occlusion of an artery. It takes a few days until enough collaterals and anastomoses are built up and sufficient blood circulation again is possible . The collateral circulation does not exclude the validity of coronary theory. Disorders of the myocardial metabolism cannot be prevented by anastomoses and collaterals. Myocardial theory is not proven by the collateral cycle.

For Bertold Kern, ouabain was the method of choice for the prevention and elimination of metabolic disorders of the heart cells in the inner layer of the left ventricle. *"Just as fire-retardant-impregnated wood is largely protected against the embers of various aetiologies, "ouabain-impregnated" myocardium also proves to be astonishingly resistant to a wide variety of interfering or destructive noxae."*

Kern assumed that ouabain protects and corrects the metabolism of the heart cell. He described ouabain as the *"most versatile broad-spectrum cardiac drug"* that is superior to all other cardiac drugs, including other cardiac glycosides. Ouabain has an *"energizing effect"* through which the heart is enabled to higher energy performances. In the case of insufficient hearts, the *energeticum effect* of ouabain remedies the insufficiency. Healthy hearts are also enabled by ouabain to perform beyond what would be possible without ouabain support. For Kern, *"the insufficient muscle fibre is chemically, structurally, etc. altered in such a way that its metabolism in the energy sector is inadequate."* Ouabain largely normalizes the functional fine structure of the myocardium. This enables not only normally sufficient, but often also abnormally high energy levels to be achieved without damage. Although Kern postulates pronounced effects of ouabain on the energy metabolism, he does not give reference to the well-known extensive literature on the metabolic effect of cardiac glycosides. He mentions the known differences between ouabain and Digitalis active ingredients on the lactic acid metabolism of the heart muscle. *"But such chemical effects are not the cause, but the result of structural normalization."*

From today's perspective, it is also incomprehensible that Kern hardly addresses the many studies on the influence of the sympathetic nervous system and its neurotransmitter, catecholamines, on the heart. He is aware of their basic effects. He mentions "stress with catecholamine-induced metabolic excess to many times the upper standard limit" in the parable of the domestic water pipe. Stress also plays a prominent role in the *pluricausal diversity* of noxae. Although the research results of Raab, Schimert, Selye and many others fit well into left myocardiology, Kern does not discuss these findings. One reason may be that these authors grant blood circulation an important role as a risk factor in the development of heart attacks, but Kern vehemently rejects this.

Kern's theses on left myocardiology have been noted with curiosity by many experts. The pharmaceutical industry was also interested in developing a product for heart attack prophylaxis based on left myocardiology and ouabain. From 1968 to 1971, Dr. Hans-Joachim Tepe, head of drug development at Tropon Werke in Cologne, had an intensive and friendly exchange of ideas with Berthold Kern on the therapeutic possibilities arising from left myocardiology. In a letter to Kern dated June 1, 1970, Tepe reported on a symposium at the Troponwerke in May 1970 at which leading cardiologists from Germany and abroad (including Bing and Raab from the USA) had dealt positively with Kern's theses. Kern's comments on prophylactic glycoside therapy should, if possible, be supported by clinical studies. The research department of Tropon Werke had already made similar statements in an assessment of the Kern theses.

Kern was initially unable to provide any experimental evidence for his hypothesis that ouabain influences the metabolism of the heart muscle. In his publications Kern does not mention the extensive research by Gremels from the 1930s as well as many relevant findings by other scientists. It was not until the collaboration with Manfred von Ardenne that Kern became aware of an experimental clue.

Manfred von Ardenne (1907 - 1997) was an award-winning scientist who made groundbreaking inventions in several fields. In addition to numerous publications and books, he has applied for more than 600 patents in radio and television technology, electron microscopy, nuclear, plasma and medical technology. His best-known inventions include the scanning electron microscope and oxygen multi-step therapy. In 1928 he founded the von Ardenne Laboratory for Electron Physics in Berlin-Lichterfelde, which he ran until 1945. After the Second World War von Ardenne was interned in the Soviet Union for ten years. In 1955 he returned to Germany and settled in Dresden.

There he was able to take over the inventory from the Lichterfelde Laboratory and received permission from the GDR government to set up a private research institute in the Dresden district "Weißer Hirsch", which bore his name and which he headed until 1990. At times, up to 500 people were employed there.

In the 1970s, von Ardenne conducted a series of studies on the resorbability of oral ouabain. In 1971 he proved that orally administered ouabain leads to short-term characteristic changes in the ECG, which can also be observed after intravenous administration, thus confirming the work of Altmann and Roth from the 1950s. In 1974, von Ardenne concluded from measurements of tritium-labelled active ingredient that ouabain was 100% absorbed after oral administration. Due to methodological errors - the tritium marking is unstable, the tritium is exchanged with other compounds - this work is of no importance. The same applies to studies in which he tries to prove a complete absorption by mathematical derivations.

Also in 1971, von Ardenne developed a micro pH glass electrode that allowed to perform pH measurements at the cellular level. The normal pH in the heart muscle tissue of rats was determined to about 7.0 with this electrode. Reduction of the blood supply to the heart by partial ligature of a coronary artery lowers the pH to about 6.4. The tissue becomes acidic. Addition of ouabain increases the pH value to the initial value. Ouabain eliminates the hyperacidity of tissue [Ardenne 1971, 1972].[10] Kern's assumption that ouabain has an effect on the metabolism of the heart muscle was thus again experimentally substantiated.

---

[10] The effect of oxygen deficiency on the acidity of the heart muscle was confirmed in 2002 by measuring isolated rabbit hearts with a specially developed electrode [Marzouk 2002]. Lack of oxygen leads to overacidification of the extracellular fluid in the heart and simultaneously increases the concentration of lactate and potassium.

The acid sensitivity of the heart muscle is well known and well documented. At pH values below 6.2, irreversible damage occurs. That is why in cardiac surgery the pH value is constantly monitored during operations [Healey 2009]. In the Strophanthin era, German surgeons routinely administered 0.3 mg of ouabain intravenously preoperatively and thus observed significantly fewer complications in heart operations.

Based on the experimental findings of Ardenne, Kern and von Ardenne have further refined left myocardiology. The myocardial infarction is a consequence of the decay of heart cells caused by acidification of the heart muscle through damage to or dissolution of the outer cell membrane (necrosis). This decay process, also known as lysomal cytolysis, is caused by special enzymes activated by acid (pH < 7) [Ardenne, Kern 1971, Ardenne 1978].

For Kern, heart muscle damage, which is associated with angina pectoris and can also lead to heart attacks, is always located in the left inner layers. They are not caused by clogged coronary arteries. Causes of left ventricle damage are myocardially damaging noxae that accumulate in the myocardium and deteriorate the performance of the heart. The left ventricle is metabolically disturbed, it gets into a state of acidosis. If the damage to the left inner layers is sufficiently advanced, a minor cause may be sufficient to increase acidosis beyond the limit of myocardial viability. At a certain pH value, myocardial death occurs, always first in small heart necroses, which expand into large necroses (infarcts). Ouabain protects the heart muscle from metabolic damage. It prevents acidification of the heart muscle and thus prevents lysomal cytolysis.

This pathogenesis of heart attack, refined by Kern and von Ardenne, received neither recognition nor attention in science. It was simply ignored. Kern's reputation - and as collateral damage that of Ardenne - was so damaged by other events that hardly any scientist was still prepared to deal with the theses of *"the Dr. Kern"*.

The Heidelberg Tribunal

Berthold Kern made intensive efforts to propagate his left myocardiology. The *Internationale Gesellschaft für Infarktbekämpfung e.V.* (International Society for Infarction Control) was founded on the occasion of the publication of his book *Der Myokardinfarkt* in 1968. It was an association of about 50 physicians who supported Kern's theses on left myocardiology with publications and events. At the same time, this society advocated oral ouabain therapy. Ouabain has been praised as the sole drug to treat metabolic disorders of the heart. Only ouabain is able to prevent acidosis of the heart muscle and the resulting necroses with subsequent infarction. Until 1970 *Strophoral* was recommended, but then the *Strodival* of Herbert GmbH was used.

Kern's theses gained nationwide attention through a series of articles in the weekly magazine *"Bunte Illustrierte"*. From 1967 to 1971, *Bunte* published several articles in which the coronary theory of heart attacks was described as a scientific error. Oral ouabain therapy based on Kern's left myocardiology has been described as the only correct treatment and prevention of heart attack.

~ ~ ~

The Bunte Illustrierte, published by Burda publishing house, had already caused a sensation several times with publications on *medical miracle cures*. In June 1961, *Bunte* reported on a discovery by the pharmacist Federico Diaz from Rivera (Uruguay) that *a new cancer treatment had been discovered*: "Lisado de Corazon". In a two-page story in *Bunte Illustrierte,* cures were reported not only for cancer, but also for other diseases such as diabetes or asthma. A few months later, the magazine published a 29-line letter in which Lisado discoverer Diaz explained that the product loses its effect just four hours after production. Therefore *testing outside of Rivera is impossible*.

In 1964, *Bunte* reported several times on an anti-cancer drug called *Bamfolin,* which *"only breaks down the pathological growths, but leaves the healthy tissue intact and has demonstrably caused cancer tumours to disappear in several people"*. Bamfolin was obtained in Japan from a certain type of bamboo grass called „*sasa*". The publisher, Dr. Franz Burda, personally took up the pen and wrote in issue 25, 1964 in the *Bunte*: *"The Japanese researchers who discovered the anticancer drug Bamfolin came to Germany. The "Bunte" reported passionlessly and factually about it. Now we receive countless calls for help every day from patients and doctors asking for Bamfolin. That's understandable. The sick reach for Bamfolin as the last straw. They seek salvation from the terrible scourge of cancer."* The German ambassador to Japan reported that Bamfolin had become a difficult problem for practically all European embassies in Tokyo. Due to the great publicity that the "Bunte Illustrierte" has made for this remedy, the ambassies are overwhelmed with numerous telephone, telegraphic and written requests for procurement - the remedy is almost unknown in Japan.

Bamfolin supporters founded societies to promote the miracle drug: the "International Bamfolin Research Community" and the "German Research Foundation for Bamfolin". But there were supply problems. It was only when a relative of a cancer patient flew to Japan and inquired locally about Bamfolin, that it became clear how and where the miracle drug was produced. *"Visited Yokoyama laundry,"* wrote the Japanese visitor. *"Sad, sad."* The miracle grass is ground up in a wooden crate, cooked with calcium hydroxide and the Bamfolin is finally extracted with the help of alcohol [SPIEGEL 1964]. Shortly thereafter, the Bamfolin companies announced:

The assessments by renowned cancer researchers from all over the world including the University of Tokyo are *devastating*. ... Bamfolin is no longer available, export from Japan blocked..." *It has not been tried, tested, or proven. It is irresponsible to put any hope in it."*

The editor-in-chief of the influential medical journal *euromed* wrote an open letter to Franz Burda published in the DIE ZEIT on August 14, 1964. It says:

> "I accuse you, Senator E. H. Dr. Franz Burda: You have irresponsibly raised false hopes for healing in thousands and thousands of cancer patients. You speculate on oral advertising, on people continuing to tell: The "Bunte" reports continuously about a new cancer cure. In fact, this rumor is already spreading all over the world. The "Bunte" did the rest to obscure the clear facts. It reported miracles, but wisely concealed the meagre Japanese results. Not even in the country of the rising Bamfolin has the drug been approved to date. ...

> "I accuse you, Senator Dr. Burda, of abusing press freedom for a mere publicity manoeuvre on your own behalf." [ZEIT 1964].

According to DER SPIEGEL, the edition of the *Bunte* increased by almost 150,000 copies during the Bamfolin campaign.

~ ~ ~

In 1967, *Bunte Illustrierte* started a series of articles on heart attacks under the lurid title "No one has to die of a heart attack". Peter Schmidsberger, Head of the science section of *Bunte* organized the campaign. Schmidsberger omitted the personal distance indispensable for a neutral journalist and made the infarct campaign his personal concern. He joined the International Society for Infarction Control. The design and style of the articles corresponded to those of the Bamfolin campaign. The coronary theory on the pathogenesis of heart attack was branded as a *heresy*. Ouabain was praised as a panacea against heart diseases and reliable protection from heart attacks:

- Sensational discovery by German doctors: protection from heart attacks (Issue 38, 1967)
- The Pill against Heart Attack (Issue 51, 1967)

- The dreaded arteriosclerosis is not the cause of heart disease. This sensational explanation is supported by convincing scientific evidence. (Issue 48, 1969)

- Treatment results on 16,000 cardiac patients within 22 years: Not a single fatal heart attack (instead of at least 130 expected under coronary measures), only 20 non-fatal heart attacks (issue 48, 1969)

- Acquittal for arteriosclerosis (Issue 39, 1971)

- I am also a victim of orthodox medicine (Issue 40, 1971)

- People suffering from infarction are the victims of a false doctrine (Issue 42, 1971).

Other newspapers adopted the topic and also reported on Kern's doctrine.

- No one needs to die of a heart attack(Stern, Issue 39, 1971)

- Nine out of ten infarct patients would not have had to die of this disease if they had been properly treated by their doctor (Welt am Sonntag, 19. 9. 1971).

- Tens of thousands of cardiac patients have been treated by Dr. Kern and his team in recent years according to myocardial theory without a fatal heart attack. (Stuttgarter Zeitung, 14. 9. 1971)

On April 28, 1970 Deutschlandfunk (a public radio station) broadcasted a lecture by Kern entitled "The prevented prevention of heart attacks". Kern massively criticized the university chairs:

"In theory, the sovereign people had long been the employer of their scientific civil servants. But only recently has it been demanded and controlled that their service may no longer suffer from unrestrained arbitrariness in opinion, claiming, denying, acting or mistreatment. Research civil servants are granted the fundamental right to freedom of opinion and teaching, inter alia, that they do not come into conflict, for the sake of their career and prestige, to have to continue to practice and teach disproved but still authoritative teachings to the detriment of the sick. Research personnel should therefore finally be spared the often discussed conflict between career and progress. For this very reason, the people have limited their scientific servants in the freedom of their opinions. So also by the duty to selflessly revoke their own outdated doctrines in the service of truth and to let all scientific progress become effective for teaching and health care. For problems of the magnitude of heart attack prevention, it becomes particularly clear how important such boundaries between what is allowed and what is forbidden would be."

The television magazine *Report* on September 13, 1971 also presented Kern's theory and oral ouabain therapy to a broad public in a programme *"In case of error death"*. Conventional medicine has been accused of failure to prevent heart attacks and disregard for the method offered by Dr. Kern: *"Heart medicine is helpless in the face of this mass death, although it could possibly prevent it."*

Orthodox medicine had to react to the massive accusations made publicly. On September 28, 1971, Prof. Gotthard Schettler wrote in a letter to the newspaper *Welt am Sonntag* :

"As President of the German Society for Internal Medicine, I cannot accept it if German internists, especially cardiologists and clinicians, are presented as malicious stubborn ignorant. I think it would be fair for the daily press to bring arguments from university professors, as Mr. Kern is now bringing them. Professor Gillmann/Ludwigshafen is concerned with exposing the core of Kern's theories. I find it almost incredible that Kern quotes the Dusseldorf clinician Edens, who never used ouabain orally, but was the expert in intravenous ouabain therapy. This is still one of the standard therapies for heart failure today. It has never been possible to eliminate heart failure by oral ouabain. I think Mr. Kern knows that too. This may be the reason why he hides or ignores this strict differentiation of intravenous and oral ouabain therapy. The well-known and high-ly respected Heidelberg clinician Fraenkel has introduced Strophanthin to the treatment of heart diseases. He would turn in his grave when he experienced this polemic."

On October 12, 1971, Berthold Kern received an invitation from the Society for Internal Medicine to a *medical discussion* as part of a public event that was to take place in Heidelberg on November 19, 1971 and at which his theses were to be discussed. Media representatives should be present at the event. Kern accepted the invitation.

On October 19, 1971, the newspaper *Giessener Allgemeine Zeitung* published an article entitled "New infarction theory - medical juggle-ry?" In it, Kern's theses were rejected by university clinicians as not verifiable. Kern should no longer refuse to engage in discussions with cardiologists, but should instead face the experts. The newspaper reported that Dr. Kern was *"invited to present his theories, which were nothing more than "immature ideas", to a competent committee in Heidelberg in November. Kern could not be taken for full, the matter was "a political attack to diminish the image of orthodox medicine".*

On October 21, 1971 Schmidsberger reacted with a letter to the *Giessener Allgemeine Zeitung*:

"Such know-it-all, which is unencumbered by any compulsion, but which is all the more highly presented from above, comes from the same corner as the request that Dr. Kern should face his opponents. Dr. Kern and the "International Society for Infarction Control" have - as usual - presented their research in scientific papers over the last twenty years. In contrast, an inquisition court is not customary, for example in the form that *recognized* doctors sit in court over colleagues who are not recognized by them according to their *dogmas*. Presumed resemblance to God is of no significance for scientific truth-finding. . ... He (Kern) was invited to a discussion and accepted this invitation. But when Dr. Kern is told by the other side within three days of receiving the letter that he is avoiding such a conversation, there are still many expectations for the future. Polemical motivations against the proponents of unpleasant ideas instead of the objective effort to coordinate opinion with facts - it would not be an isolated case in the history of medicine".

Schmidsberger and Kern knew that the event in Heidelberg would hardly be a scientific discussion. They had to prepare for a public hearing. An agreement was reached according to which a representative of the Society for Internal Medicine and a representative of the Society for Infarction Control would alternately chair the discussions.

On October 28, 1971, the statement by Prof. Gillmann announced by Schettler in the letter to the Welt am Sonntag appeared in *Deutsches Ärzte Blatt* [Gillmann 1971]. Therein Gillmann criticizes the style of Kern's depictions:

> "One may hope that at least the exaggerated formulations are not in the sense of the doctor Kern, but journalistic "hangers". Kern must be aware, however, that his provocative formulations almost provoke the representatives of the lay press to bring them as a gag - preferably with sequels.
>
> However, it is about more than the style of debate among doctors: The representations described above and directed to the layperson are ultimately at the expense of our patients. Instead of taking advantage of the numerous possibilities of discussion at congresses and symposia, the at least tolerated provocative presentation on television provides the layman and the patient with information that makes him doubt not only about medical science but also about his doctor. ...
>
> I have therefore agreed to prepare this commentary despite some reservations. The concerns are based on the fact that it is difficult to comment with facts on a doctrine that at least seems to correspond more to a doctrine of faith with discipleship than to a self-critical science. Possibly the rejection by

"orthodox medicine" has also contributed to the fixation of this attitude."

Gillmann denies that orthodox medicine officially regards the clogging of the coronary vessels as the sole cause of the heart attack. Referring to his textbook, he points out that an imbalance between oxygen supply and oxygen demand is decisive. This imbalance is influenced by many factors. A complete occlusion of the vessel is not a prerequisite for a heart attack, as it is always a balance problem. Only a certain relative reduction in blood flow must be achieved, which triggers the local chain reaction. The situation at the myocardial cell is decisive. Here the view of orthodox medicine coincides with that of Kern. Differences, however, would exist in the view of the significance. Kern prioritizes the metabolism of the myocardial cell, the orthodox medicine the circulatory disorder. The increasing importance of beta receptor blockers, which, in addition to limiting excessive adrenergic reactions, are aimed at regulating the heart rate, indicates a change in attitudes.

Gillmann is much more critical of Kern's statements on the success rate of oral ouabain therapy. It is known that oral ouabain has a very low bioavailability and is unreliable. Kern's success statistics are not comprehensible and not documented according to scientific standards. *"In contrast to Kern, however, none of the scientifically oriented self-critical doctors feels able to claim that he has found the therapy in which no one needs to die of a heart attack."* Gillmann expresses the opinion that *"only a debate in an emotionally unburdened atmosphere makes it possible to clarify positions"*.

~ ~ ~

The "medical discussion", held at the invitation of the Society for Internal Medicine, took place on November 19, 1971 in the Molkenkur Restaurant, located above Heidelberg near Heidelberg Castle. More than 150 people were present, including 25 members of the Society for Infarction Control. The mood was frosty and, unlike Gillmann wanted, emotionally charged. Prof. Wollheim from Würzburg refused to share the chairmanship of the meeting with a representative of the Society for Infarction Control as agreed. He alone chaired the meeting and determined who was allowed to speak on which topic and when. Contributions by representatives of Kern's myocardial theory were hardly considered. Kern was not allowed to comment on the reproaches, but was urged to answer "yes" or "no". Several times he was ultimately asked to revoke his theses. It was a medieval Inquisition procedure. Wollheim was prosecutor and judge in one person. The accused Berthold Kern was the subject of the trial. He had no legal hearing, as an accused is entitled to as a party to the trial before a court. His participation in the show trial took place only insofar as this was necessary for the formal determination of a previously determined judgement.

Kern's negligence in presenting his own hypotheses as facts considerably weakened his position. Several times he had first correctly formulated circumstances as hypotheses and later transformed them into factual assertions without any evidence. Initially, Kern merely postulated complete absorption of ouabain after oral administration. Over the years, he then described the complete absorption as a fact. He was unable to present any measurement data for this in Heidelberg. From published observations on the absorption and excretion of ouabain in cats, Kern had derived the hypothesis that even doses of 80 mg within 24 hours of slow injection would have no effect in humans. Although it was known that doses of more than 1 mg lead to *Strophanthin death*, he described this postulate as a fact in his book *The Myocardial Infarction*. In the Heidelberg Tribunal he then had to reveal that he had merely estimated this information mathematically, but never determined it experimentally. Kern's claim that his ouabain-treated patients had no heart attacks was limited to observations while the patients had been in his treatment. He had no information on the fate of patients who had changed to other doctors or stopped treatment because of dissatisfaction with his therapy.

The invited representatives of orthodox medicine emphasized the central importance of coronary blood flow and coronary thrombosis

126

for the development of heart attacks. Organic diseases of the coronary arteries are responsible for all heart attacks. Kern's statements to the contrary cannot be supported by scientifically accepted facts.

Kern's recommended infarction prophylaxis with oral ouabain was dismissed as nonsense. It is known how unreliable oral ouabain is and even the proven low bioavailability would speak against an effect. Kern's claim that he had not observed a heart attack after oral ouabain treatment in more than 16,000 patients in his practice was dismissed as implausible. The patient data were not scientifically correct evaluated. *"Mr. Kern, no one will believe that you have not had a heart attack death among your clientele."* As in the times of the Strophoral dispute, it was denied that the patients treated by Kern had suffered from heart disease. Prof. Beyer, Berlin: *"We see that there is not a single symptom in Kern's symptoms that would justify the assumption of angina pectoris disease. ... I believe that the reason for the different statistics lies in the completely different composition of the medical goods. Send me the 16,000, I'll evaluate them in four weeks and tell you who had what and who didn't!"* As von Schmiedeberg postulated in the second half of the 19th century, orthodox physicians denied that there were differences in the effects of ouabain and Digitalis agents. Prof. Kuschinsky: *"There is absolutely no experimental evidence that ouabain or other cardiac glycosides have a different effect on the muscles of the left and right ventricle".* The accusation of maltreatment with Digitalis was vigorously protested. Prof. Heinecker: *"We other doctors who do not treat according to Kern's recommendations are massively accused of wrongly treating our angina pectoris patients and our infarct patients. We are threatened with the prosecutor that we will not treat with oral ouabain because we are such narrow-minded orthodox physicians. Who speaks of the public prosecutor in patients who for years were very well adjusted to Digitalis and now get oral ouabain and come to us in the clinic with pulmonary edema?"*

Here, too, Kern is urged to revoke his theses. Prof. Gillmann: *"Mr. Kern, at least tell us once, I think that everyone is waiting for you to have to back off in certain things that you have claimed. Why don't you admit that what you say: that Digitalis therapy is wrong, even triggers a heart attack, and that oral ouabain therapy alone is correct - that you take it back"* and continued: *"The question about the prosecutor, Dr. Kern, must be clarified!"* When Kern did not respond to these reproaches, Wollheim terminated the conference: *"What Mr. Gillmann says, Dr. Kern, is a very serious matter. It cannot remain unchallenged that all of us who do not use such a treatment with oral ouabain commit a crime or act unscrupulously. That's not possible."*

There was only one point on which everyone involved agreed: A comprehensive clinical examination of oral ouabain therapy is necessary to confirm or refute Kern's theses. But Prof. Schettler consistently blocked this proposal with his closing remarks:

> "It all seems to be that we are now being asked to cooperate and offered to start new investigations in a variety of sectors. Everything that has been written in recent months is untrue today. Under these circumstances, I would now ask you to read the text of the lecture on Deutschlandfunk radio, where personal attacks against representatives of orthodox medicine in a variety of areas have been launched in such a way that one simply no longer can follow. If it is assumed that a German doctor, if he is full professor, can claim today what he wants, he would never be reprimanded for it, he would never be held accountable for it, if it is further written that the expert opinions, which are provided by us, are to the detriment of patients out of arrogance and ignorance of orthodox medicine, and if these things are quoted as proof of a miserable performance of this so-called orthodox medicine, if the whole thing is still dressed up politically - ladies and gentlemen, I personally, as a doctor with all my commitment, can no longer be involved!"

The day after the tribunal, a press conference was held at which a paper prepared solely by the Society for Internal Medicine was distributed as *Results of the scientific colloquium on the theses of Dr. Kern on November 19, 1971.* The report also criticized Ardenne's work on lysomal cytolysis as not scientifically proven. This research had not been mentioned or discussed the day before. A clear indication that the final communique had already been formulated before the beginning of the "medical discussion". The paper denied the effects of oral ouabain therapy:

"The key point is the assertion that approximately 100,000 patients have been saved from a heart attack by oral ouabain treatment and that this treatment is a hundred percent prevention of heart attack. Second attacks would also be practically prevented by such treatment.

In the view of the discussion participants, these claims can only be proven if appropriate scientific documentation is provided. However, the publications of Dr. Kern and his working group only contain information that does not in any way correspond to the generally accepted principles of medical statistics. This applies both to the documentation of the cases and to the evaluation of the allegedly recorded patient pool. Prevention and treatment of heart attacks, especially the numerous primary and secondary preventive studies carried out all over the world, are not taken into account by Dr. Kern either in his documentation or in his theories. It is outrageous that Dr. Kern bases his blanket assertions on such inadequate documentation.

On the basis of the findings available and discussed so far, the material and the presentation by Dr. Kern, it cannot be claimed that his therapy prevents heart attacks. According to all available evidence, such an assertion is unjustified."

Finally, the document of the Society for Internal Medicine concluded

"The scientists present are of the opinion that it is irresponsible for Dr. Kern's theses to be further disseminated to the public before their truth has been sufficiently proven by a prospective, controlled investigation."

The communique of the Society for Internal Medicine was published in *Deutsches Medizinisches Journal*, Issue 2, 1972. The medical journal "euromed" also published it in full. On December 14, 1971 Schmidsberger wrote to a friend in the USA: *"An angry tribunal has now met here. Eighty "authorities" have torn Dr. Kern apart. He has made an impossible figure tactically and rhetorically. His opponents had it easy, we've had it hard ever since."*

The response to the Heidelberg Tribunal was unanimous: Dr. Kern's theses have been refuted. DER SPIEGEL called Kern's theses *humbug* and *closed madness system* [Spiegel 1971]. On March 20, 1972, the specialist journal "selecta" reported on *gutted infarct theses*: *"He who leaves the soil of medicine and its scientific foundations is a witchdoctor. He should be characterized by an adequate number of feathers."* ZDF, a public tv-station, ended a report on the Heidelberg event on November 22, 1971 with the statement *"Dr. Kern was scientifically disqualified"*.

Peter Schmidsberger documented his perception of the Heidelberg Tribunal in the book *Skandal Herzinfarkt* (Scandal Heart Attack*)*. Therein he claims the sole correctness of myocardial theory. Coronary theory is based on proven false dogmas [Schmidsberger 1975]. He intended to present the book at the 1975 annual meeting of the Society for Infarction Control in Stuttgart. But the Society for Infarction Control rejected the suggestion. They did not want to identify with the book. The public discussion had already failed once. The campaign of the *Bunte Illustrierte* only hurt. They did not want to upset the doctors again. It was therefore not possible to present the book during the congress in Stuttgart.

In a letter dated March 6, 1975, Schmidsberger complained to Kern about the decision of the Gesellschaft für Infarktbekämpfung (IGI): *"I respect this attitude and will act accordingly. If the IGI is so distinguished that my public relations work is not enough for it, I would at least like to remind you that without our efforts the discussion about heart attacks would still be in the Stone Age. It is also ridiculous to believe that the public, and above all the teaching medicine, will keep apart the book "Scandal Heart Attack" and the group around Kern (the IGI is nothing more than a support organization for your life's work). They will have no more than a tired smile for any distancing. What miracle workers and dream dancers am I dealing with?"* Schmidsberger angrily left the Society for Infarction Control.

Schmidsberger was not a journalist who reported neutrally on a matter. He was actively involved in the discussion of Kern's theses and had controlled the infarct campaign of the *Bunte Illustrierte* to increase the circulation from the very beginning. He has also influenced Berthold Kern in many ways:

Berthold Kern fought for the right knowledge, the truth, without alternative. Nature observation, logic and consistent thinking had led him to *left myocardiology*. Therefore, there could be no doubt about his theses. He relentlessly branded even minor inconsistencies in the statements of others. Even proponents of ouabain therapy were not exempt. Prof. Sarre, Freiburg, had shown in clinical studies in the 1950s that oral ouabain significantly eases symptoms in angina pectoris patients while Digitalis agents worsen the condition of patients. Although oral ouabain was officially considered ineffective after the Heidelberg Tribunal, Sarre reaffirmed his commitment to his studies at the end of 1971. Kern criticized Sarre for still arguing on the basis of coronary theory. In a letter dated January 19, 1972 Schmidsberger expressed his displeasure at Kern's behavior:

> "The Sarre Brief is a true joy. Not only does he fully acknowledge his work, he also distinguishes between utilisation disorder and heart failure, he points to the qualitative difference between Digitalis and ouabain, and to the necessary distinction between inotropic and oxygen-using effects of Digitalis and ouabain.
>
> But your answer to Sarre is all the more unpleasant. With this tactic and such formulations you will not win supporters, but on the contrary, even those who are on the same line will be offended. May I quote some passages?

You call coronary insufficiency theory "questionable" and "erroneous". In the same context, however, you find that it is "the same so-called coronary insufficiency that you see as the mental basis... on which they were based." So you're telling a scientist whom you want to win for yourself that he has a mental concept like a jerk. Couldn't you phrase something like that more elegantly?

And further in the text: "Recently I recommend clinicians who are still bound to the imaginary world of coronary insufficiency..." Or even: "The spiritual bridge is usually not recognized...". Don't you notice that here too you correspond with a clinician who is still bound to the concept of coronary insufficiency? Do you think he's interested in letting you "recommend" something to him? Or do you think he's particularly happy to hear from you that he's too stupid to see a spiritual bridge?

And why is the first thing you have to bang around someone else's ears the nonsense of coronary theory? ...

It certainly annoys others when they always come across formulations such as: "More in my book on heart attacks" - "which we have worked out since 1947 and published since 1948" - "for other reasons which I have often published" - "compare my monograph "Herzinsuffizienz". For once you are resented for quoting yourself instead of formulating. On the other hand, nobody is curious about what you published first and when.

Dear Mr. Kern, these are rather harsh words. But now you simply have to subordinate yourself to a tactical route that may not be yours. For the coming months, you, the spiritual forefather of this whole topic, have nothing more to be than an informer who himself remains completely in the background. Any emphasis on one's own performance is completely inappropriate and only prevents the breakthrough of your concerns."

This letter not only clarifies Berthold Kern's style of argumentation. It also illustrates the strong influence Schmidsberger exerted on Kern in the infarct campaign of the *Bunte Illustrierte* and in the resulting disputes with orthodox medicine.

After the Heidelberg Tribunal, Berthold Kern was hardly noticed by orthodox medicine any more. He continued to advocate his theses, but increasingly shifted his work to epistemological questions. He drew no discernible lessons from his experiences in the disputes with orthodox medicine on left-heart failure, the Strophoral dispute and on left myocardiology. He held on to his search for the pure truth and was ready to fight for it. On March 8, 1975 he wrote to Schmidsberger:

"Since Heidelberg" it has become increasingly clear to me that one cannot progress on the path of gentle whispering or even change your opponents mind. But since the beginnings and stormy developments of epistemology it has become clear to me that there is nothing else to do but to openly reveal the wrongdoings of the incorrigible malfunction and to acknowledge them as irreversible, with clarification also of the appalling consequences for the public, which tolerates and finances this kind of unscience in place of the required science. This direction was taken by you in the Scandal Book, and the same direction is taken in my treatises."

The Medicines Act

After the Heidelberg Tribunal, orally administered ouabain was considered a medical malpractice by orthodox physicians. Ernst Eden's prophecy that the omission of ouabain treatment would one day be classified as a medical malpractice had been turned to the contrary. Schettler formulated in 1977:

> "If the proponents of the sublingual use of ouabain claim that their findings are irresponsibly attacked and combated to the detriment of patients, it should be noted that ouabain solutions for sublingual or oral administration are available on the drug market in Germany, unlike in other countries, and that every doctor is free to decide whether or not to use them. However, in the case of a therapy trial, every physician should be aware that the oral or perlingual administration of ouabain is neither a theoretically justified nor an empirically proven or at least probably effective treatment method." [Schettler 1977].

Erland Erdmann, cardiologist at the University of Munich, went even further. He also rejected intravenous Strophanthin therapy: "Accordingly, there is no longer a reliable indication for Strophanthin, whether orally, perlingually or intravenously [Erdmann 1985]. Even the generally accepted clinical experiences of Fraenkel and Edens with intravenous Strophanthin therapy were sacrificed to the *medical Zeitgeist*. Scientific journals also dissociated themselves from Strophanthin. When Salz and Schneider published the results of a small double-blind study with oral ouabain in 1985 in the *Zeitschrift für Allgemeinmedizin* [Salz 1985] the article was given a note by the editor stating that the editorial staff did not identify with the content of the article.

With this broad rejection, the decline of oral ouabain therapy had been initiated. Fewer and fewer doctors were prepared to oppose the official doctrine. In his book "Der Schlüssel zur Infarktverhütung" (The key to infarct prevention) H. Christophersen quotes an unnamed research director of a large pharmaceutical company, who aptly describes the situation of ouabain according to the Heidelberg Tribunal: "We would immediately bring out Strophanthin in a big way if we could conceal its real name. The name Strophanthin has been discredited too much in recent decades. Only when g-Strophanthin has been rehabilitated all over the world can we change our position." [Christophersen 1973].

The decline of ouabain therapy was accelerated by the enactment of the Medicines Act. Until 1961, Germany did not have its own drug law regulating the marketing of drugs. A pharmaceutical act was enacted in Germany in 1961 as a condition of the EU Treaties of Rome. Initially, it only regulated the registration of substances *"whose efficacy was not generally known"*. It did not contain any obligation to test the efficacy and safety of the drugs, but only envisaged a registration. When using substances whose efficacy is not *"generally known"*, a report on the nature and extent of observed side effects should be included.

From 1964 the testing of the drugs was prescribed by pre-clinical and clinical studies. The manufacturers of medicines had to give a written assurance that the medicine had been sufficiently and carefully tested in accordance with the current state of scientific knowledge. In 1971, binding principles for the pharmacological-toxicological and clinical testing of pharmaceuticals were established. Only drugs that had been tested according to these guidelines were approved. The thalidomide scandal then prompted a fundamental redesign of the Medicines Act to improve drug safety in order to protect patients.

The drug *Contergan* was a tranquilizer containing the active ingredient thalidomide. Until the end of the 1950s, it was recommended as a non-prescription sedative and sleeping pill for pregnant women. When taken during early pregnancy, severe malformations and sometimes also the lack of limbs and organs in newborns occurred. Worldwide, several thousand children were born injured by thalidomide. In addition, there was an unknown number of stillbirths. At the end of 1961, the connection between thalidomide and the malformations was recognised and the drug was taken off the market by the manufacturer, Grünenthal GmbH in Stolberg. The scandal had a worldwide impact on the practice of drug approvals.

After years of consulting, a completely new drug law was passed in Germany in 1976. Since then, the approval procedure for a drug has had to prove its quality, efficacy and safety. Be required:

- a dossier on the pharmaceutical quality of the preparation

- pharmacological and toxicological studies and

- clinical studies to prove safety and efficacy

Medicines that were already on the market before 1978 were classified as "fictitiously approved". Manufacturers were required to demonstrate the safety and efficacy of their products within a generous transition period of 12 years by means of appropriate studies („subsequent approval"). The implementation of these legal requirements was handled generously. A large number of registrations had not yet been completed in 1997. The "fictitious approvals" were renewed. Companies that had not submitted any safety and efficacy studies by the reporting date on February 1, 2001 have lost their product approvals. The companies had the right - with the possibility of a final sales period of up to 2.5 years - to waive their approval beforehand. As a result of this regulation, around 10,000 approvals expired in Germany in 2001. But even this period had been extended again in many cases. The required studies for numerous "fictitious approvals" had not yet been submitted in Germany at the end of 2004. The EU Commission then instituted infringement proceedings against the Federal Republic of Germany. In the procedure, the Federal Government undertook to complete the processing of applications for subsequent approval by the end of 2005.

The requirements of the Medicines Act also applied to the ouabain preparations on the market, as they did to all other existing drugs.

Almost all remaining manufacturers of ouabain-based products were medium-sized companies that were unable to finance the required studies. Several companies also contacted Kern and the Society for Infarction Control with a request for support. In 1985, in a "Strophanthin Report," the latter again presented a paper in which the contradictoriness of coronary theory is emphasized and the sole validity of myocardial theory is claimed. Dr. Herrmann, head of the scientific department of the Strodival manufacturer Herbert GmbH, describes the situation of his company in his reaction to the Strophanthin Report in a letter to the Gesellschaft für Infarktbekämpfung on September 2, 1985:

"As manufacturer and head of the scientific department of Herbert, it is my top priority to ensure that the Strodival preparations receive final approval from the Federal Health Office (at present only a fictitious approval exists) by the end of 1989. If this does not succeed, the preparations will no longer be on the market in the 1990s.

Under these circumstances, you will understand that all my efforts are aimed at fulfilling the orthodox medical criteria of the amended Medicines Act of 1976, which also require significant statements about effects and efficacy.

Philosophical considerations about the paradigm shift in medical education, which in my opinion is long overdue, do not help me. Nor does the company Herbert have the power of assertiveness nor the necessary funds to conduct spectacular trials with any medical administrations right down to the last legal instance, especially since they can refer to the unquestionable factual material of the amended Medicines Act of 1976, whether they like it or not, and will therefore always be among the winners.

Since Dr. Kern's left myocardiology can and will only gain recognition through the orthodox acceptance of oral ouabain therapy, everything that could damage the delicate ouabain plant should be avoided in the interest of Dr. Kern's life's work. This includes, as sorry as I am to have to say this, your report."

History repeats itself. In 1951 Boehringer Mannheim asked Berthold Kern to refrain from publishing his book *Die orale Strophanthinbehandlung* with the attacks on orthodox medicine contained therein in order not to endanger the market success of Strophoral. Kern had insisted on publishing the book and thus fired the Strophoral dispute. The International Society for Infarction Control could not be dissuaded from the publication of the Strophanthin Report and thus confirmed the prejudice of the orthodox physicians to "correspond more to a doctrine of faith with discipleship than to a self-critical science". Strodival and Herbert were not helped with this publication. Herbert had to deal with new competitors.

In the 1980s, major pharmaceutical companies launched beta-blockers and ACE inhibitors with new active principles. These were propagated with the concentrated marketing power of large companies and very quickly found a high level of acceptance among doctors. Almost all ouabain providers stopped marketing their products for economic reasons. The Strodival from Herbert Arzneimittel GmbH was the only product still offered. Herbert Arzneimittel GmbH was acquired in 1996 by Brahms Arzneimittel AG, which was acquired by the Swedish generics manufacturer Meda in 2003. In 2016 Meda was acquired by Mylan Pharmaceuticals. Meda has also not carried out any of the studies necessary for Strodival's subsequent approval. As a generics company Meda does not develop new drugs. The company confines itself to the manufacture and sale of off-patent drugs. Meda had the Strodival preparations manufactured externally on a contract basis by Jäger GmbH in Muggensturm in the Black Forest. No internal Meda resources have been allocated to Strodival.

At the end of 2005, the fictitious approval for Strodival threatened to expire. A group of doctors, alternative practitioners and patients intervened with the Federal Ministry of Health and the political parties represented in the Bundestag with the aim of extending the deadline.

The BfArM (Federal Institute for Drugs and Medical Devices) then extended the fictitious approval of Strodival for the last time in agreement with the Ministry of Health with the condition that the necessary studies on the safety and effect of the product be submitted by July 2011. Meda has not provided the requested data. On July 15, 2011, the BfArM therefore withdrew the fictitious approval of Strodival. Meda was allowed to sell the Strodival stocks already produced and officially discontinued distribution on August 1, 2012. Since then, no marketable Strophanthin preparation has been available worldwide.

Strophanthin based preparations are now only available as over-the-counter homeopathic products and as prescription Defekturarzneimittel[11]. Standardized extracts of Strophanthus seeds, aqueous-alcoholic solutions of the active ingredient and solid active ingredient filled into capsules are used. None of these preparations is galenically optimized, so absorption and effect of these preparations are correspondingly uncertain.

Dr. Klaus-Dieter Beller, physician from Kenzingen, has developed a promising approach. He applies k-Strophanthin solutions with a specially developed spray technique. The dosages correspond to those of the historically proven iv application. The therapeutic successes achieved with this method on individual patients are impressive.

A lively activist scene has also established itself on the internet, propagating Strophantin preparations with irresponsible promises of salvation ("Those who regularly receive Strophanthin no longer die of heart failure.") for the treatment of a broad spectrum of sensibilities. Strophanthin is portrayed as a victim of criminal conspiracy by orthodox medicine and the pharmaceutical industry. Books on Strophanthin suggest that marketing interests of large pharmaceutical compa-

---

[11] Defekturarzneimittel are drugs that are manufactured in quantities of up to one hundred packages per day in pharmacies themselves, without requiring a manufacturing permit or drug approval in accordance with the German Medicines Act.

nies and the associated medical lobby deny and suppress the blessed Strophanthin. The absurd conspiracy theories are enriched with unconventional interpretations of experimental and clinical results. Free of any expertise, the false assertion is made that Strophanthin is found in Foxglove (!), lilies of the valley and sea onions. Although there are no current clinical studies on the efficacy of Strophanthin, it is falsely claimed that "*New studies show that Strophanthin makes expensive statins and beta-blockers superfluous.*" The Jim Humble sect has also taken over Strophanthin. This dubious organization advertises chloric acid - known as "Miracle Mineral Supplements" (MMS) - as a universal remedy against cancer, AIDS, malaria and other diseases. Such polemical and senseless activities strengthen the rejection by orthodox medicine and lead to the stigmatisation of Strophanthin as a homeopathic quack doctor's preparation.

Endogenous Ouabain

Until well into the 1950s, scientific literature hardly differentiated between k-Strophanthin and g-Strophanthin. The term "Strophanthin" was used for all cardiac glycosides derived from Strophanthus species. The g-Strophanthin isolated from Strophanthus gratus, which was used in oral and iv-Strophanthin therapy, is identical to the active ingredient ouabain isolated from Acokanthera ouabaio. In the scientific literature today, only the term "ouabain" is used for g-Strophanthin. Therefore, in the following chapters, the term "ouabain" is used to describe current results of g-Strophanthin research. The term "Strophanthin" is retained for k-Strophanthin.

~ ~ ~

Ouabain has fallen victim to the dogmatic dispute between coronary theory and myocardial theory. Its therapeutic effect is not linked to any theory with which scientists explain the pathogenesis of heart attacks. The therapeutic effect of ouabain is based on its chemical structure, which determines its pharmacological and physiological effects. After 1990, ouabain no longer played a role in the therapy of heart diseases. Meda's sales of Strodival products were in the order of less than five million euros per year. Outside Germany it was hardly known that ouabain had been used as a drug.

In pharmacological research, ouabain is used to investigate the manifold functions of the sodium pump (Na/K-ATPase). The sodium pump is an omnipresent membrane-bound enzyme, it is is involved in many physiological processes. It transports sodium ions from the cell and potassium ions into the cell. It thus ensures the vital ion gradient between the interior of cells and the extracellular fluid. The energy required for its function is obtained by hydrolysis of adenosine triphosphate. In high concentrations, Digitalis glycosides (digoxin, digitoxin) and Strophanthus glycosides (ouabain, k-Strophanthin) inhibit the sodium pump. Ouabain is used specifically to inhibit the sodium pump in experimental studies on the function of the Na/K-ATPase.

In stark contrast to decades of positive clinical experiences with ouabain in humans, in current research reports several disease states are reported to be associated with elevated levels of a compound that is claimed to be "endogenous ouabain" (EO). It has been asserted that ouabain is a key factor not only in the pathogenesis of hypertension and heart failure but in many common diseases. It is suggested that EO acts as a pro-hypertrophic and growth-promoting hormone, which might lead to cardiac remodeling affecting cardiovascular functions and structures [Blaustein 2018, Simonini 2018].

The concept of "endogenous ouabain" (EO) originated in the late 1970s when it was postulated that an endogenous inhibitor of vascular Na/K-ATPase might be a natriuretic hormone (NH) causing hypertension [Buckalew 2015]. Because of the suggestion that NH might be an inhibitor of Na/K-ATPase, it was subsequently referred to as "ouabain-like" or "Digitalis-like."

Immunoassay

The body's immune system recognizes invading foreign proteins and neutralizes them by forming highly specific defence substances (antibodies). This mechanism is used in immunoassays. Chemical compounds that one wants to detect - for example ouabain - are chemically linked to a foreign protein. This protein linked to the ouabain is injected into mice, which then form an antibody specific for this modified protein. This is isolated and used to determine ouabain in human serum. The basic problem with this method is that it is often not sufficiently specific. It also recognizes compounds that have structural similarities to the compound to be detected, but are not identical to it. False-positive results are obtained. The advantage of this method is the high sensitivity. Extremely low concentrations can be determined.

By using radioimmunoassays (RIA) based on digoxin or ouabain antibodies numerous compounds have been identified in mammalian plasma, including steroids, lipids, peptides, and a variety of other compounds [Wechter 1990]. Antibody based RIA are often subject to cross reactivity with compounds other than those to which the antibody was raised. A recent example is ionotropin. This substance has been isolated from mammalian tissue. It cross reacts with digoxin-specific antibodies, but has a proposed chemical structure that is not related to digoxin [Chasalow 2018].

It is important to note that the EO concept, in contrast to clinical experience, suggests that digoxin and ouabain as inhibitors of the Na/K-ATPase increase blood pressure. However, in more than two centuries of clinical use with therapeutic concentrations of digoxin and ouabain no hypertensinogenic effects have been observed. In clinical experience a reduction of high blood pressure in patients is observed especially on treatment with ouabain [Fürstenwerth 2015]. Already Thomas Fraser, who in cooperation with Burroughs, Wellcome & Co in 1886 had introduced a Strophanthus extract for the treatment of heart diseases, had pointed out that "*strophanthin increases the action of the heart without raising blood pressure.*" In 1908 Fraenkel had confirmed this observation by investigating the effect of Strophantus tinctures on the blood pressure and pulse of healthy people [Fraenkel 1908]. Blood pressure did not rise after application of Strophanthin.

In 1991, Hamlyn et al. together with scientists from Upjohn Laboratories in Kalamazoo, Michigan reported purification of a compound from 300 l of human plasma indistinguishable from ouabain by mass spectroscopy [Hamlyn 1991]. Thus, the decades-long search for an endogenous inhibitor of the ubiquitous sodium pump seemed to have come to a successful conclusion. The renowned scientific journal *Lancet* dedicated an editorial entitled "Welcome to Ouabain - a New Steroid Hormone" to this breakthrough. Based on this discovery, Du Pont-New England Nuclear developed a commercial immunoassay.

Subsequent work seemed to confirm this observation and indicated that mammalian ouabain is present in multiple body fluids and tissues. Numerous research groups used this detection method to determine ouabain plasma levels. The concentrations varied from "undetectable" to 2.5 ± 0.5 nmol/L to 176 ± 68 nmol/L.

Based on the hypothesis that ouabain causes hypertension the research group at the University of Maryland in cooperation with the Italian pharmaceutical company Sigma-Tau developed an ouabain antagonist that in animal model lowers blood pressure. This drug candidate was ineffective in clinical trials in humans. It showed no blood pressure lowering effect at all [Staessen 2011].

The discovery that ouabain could be an endogenous hormone renewed scientific interest in this molecule as a potentially important hormone in normal physiology and in diseases. Intensive research on possible mechanisms of action of the ouabain led to a flood of new findings. It is now believed that low concentrations of ouabain induce signaling cascades via the sodium pump that regulate a variety of cell functions, including cell proliferation (formation of new cells), hypertrophy, apoptosis (programmed cell death), metabolism and cell mobility. These effects are independent of the transport of sodium and potassium ions by the sodium pump [Silva 2012].

A series of recent experimental in-vitro and in-vivo studies with ouabain indicate cardio-protective effects and thus confirm decades of positive clinical experiences with ouabain. Ouabain prevents hypertrophy of the heart and the adrenal cortex in rats exposed to hypoxia induced by extreme exercise. In rat and rabbit hearts short exposure to a low concentration of ouabain protects the heart against ischemia/reperfusion injury. Current reports confirm cardio protection induced by ouabain [Wu 2015, Buzaglo 2018, Marck 2018]. It is suggested that ouabain can be beneficial to various stages of heart failure [Liu 2016]. In addition, experimental results indicate promising effects of ouabain in cancer and protection of kidney development from adverse effects of malnutrition [Li 2010, Khodus 2011].

The mutually exclusive effects of ouabain and the inhibitor of the Na/K-ATPase observed by radioimmunoassays in mammalian tissues

do not support the hypothesis that this inhibitor is identical with ouabain, but favor the interpretation that the sought after natriuretic hormone is something different, which also reacts to ouabain antibodies.

In the euphoria about the manifold new results, reports from some
working groups that no endogenous ouabain could be detected in human plasma with the help of chromatographic methods were initially
ignored. Recent work, however, casts substantial doubts on the existence of endogenous ouabain.

Vogeser et al established a stable-isotope dilution API-MS/MS method for the quantification of ouabain in human plasma [Baecher
2014]. This team developed a method of extremely high sensitivity
detecting spiked ouabain in human plasma. The method was fully
validated according to FDA guidelines and published in the official
journal of the International Federation of Clinical Chemistry after
peer review. Using this method, no ouabain could be detected within
the calibration range of the method (1.7–172 pmol/l) in unspiked human plasma samples that contained EO levels of 206–665 pmol/l as
determined by radioimmunoassays in the laboratory of Paolo Manunta in Italy. So in samples of human plasma that contained considerable levels of "endogenous ouabain" as detected by radioimmunoassay, API-MS/MS based analysis did not detect any ouabain. These
results confirm the conclusions drawn from the clinical experiences
outlined in this book: endogenous ouabain is different from ouabain.
There is no ouabain in human plasma. Thus the hypothesis of endogenous ouabain is refuted.

Decades of clinical experience with ouabain provide a yardstick by
which all research results and hypotheses related to ouabain have to
be measured. Observations at the bedside are more meaningful than
speculative hypotheses based on experimental research. It is remarka-
ble that in almost all work on endogenous ouabain no reference is
made to the long-term use of ouabain and related glycosides (k-
Strophanthin, Cymarin, Convallatoxin) in the therapy of heart diseases. This part of the history of the ouabain is almost unknown in
science today. It is totally incomprehensible why nearly all scientists

involved in ouabain research do not mention the well-documented clinical experiences with ouabain in their publications.

Even worse, Mordecai P. Blaustein, Baltimore, Paolo Manunta, Milano, Italy, and John Hamlyn, Baltimore, who all fiercely advocate the existence of endogenous ouabain, not only persistently neglect the well-documented therapeutic experiences with ouabain in humans but even deny the analytical results of the Vogeser group. With dubious claims and even unfounded accusations ("edited their raw data", "scientific misconduct") it is tried to discredit Vogeser's method.

Science is a set of methods aimed at building a testable body of knowledge open to rejection or confirmation. Such an understanding of science should also form the basis in research on ouabain. Hubris and personal vanity will hinder finding the truth, but they can not stop it. In the end, truth does prevail.

Ouabain and its effects

Cardiac glycosides have been used for more than 200 years in the treatment of heart failure. Their use in clinical practice has declined sharply since the introduction of beta blockers and ACE inhibitors. Today, only the Digitalis derivatives digoxin and digitoxin are used. The guidelines for the treatment of heart failure generally recommend only supportive use of these agents in addition to beta-blockers and ACE inhibitors. But even these recommendations are not uncontroversial. Observational studies are repeatedly published in which the efficacy of these preparations is questioned. Observational studies document the effects of drugs on patients. It is not compared with patients who receive no medication or medication other than the one tested. The informative value of such studies is low [Cole 2015, de Boer 2015]. The discussion is correspondingly controversial. Comparative studies or double-blind studies have not yet been conducted for cost reasons. Manufacturers of Digitalis do not see themselves in a position to finance such studies.

Some leading cardiologists even plead for a stronger consideration of digoxin in the medical practice. They advocate a re-evaluation of the current role of Digitalis in the treatment of heart failure [Adams 2014, Ambrosy 2014]. They see an urgent need for more effective means of treating heart failure. Heart failure is the only disease whose incidence and prevalence are steadily increasing in most developed countries. Despite modern treatment with beta-blockade and full angiotensin II modulation, the five-year mortality rate of heart failure is over 50% and corresponds to that of cancer. The efficacy of today's standard medication for the treatment of heart failure in absolute terms is only a few percentage points better than placebo [Granger 2006]. In addition, it has been shown that there is a strong correlation between digoxin serum concentration and the safety and efficacy of digoxin. It is appropriate to call into question the usual dosages. Positive effects are particularly evident at serum concentrations below 1 ng/ml. The effects of digoxin at serum concentrations greater than 1 ng/ml, which have been achieved with the dosages commonly used up to now, are less advantageous. In their evaluations of all available studies, the scientists conclude that low-dose digoxin reduces the risk of hospital admissions and improves the symptoms of chronic heart failure.

Ouabain is no longer included in the discussion about the use of cardiac glycosides in the treatment of heart disease. Its use as a drug is hardly known outside Germany. In textbooks of medicine, ouabain is no longer mentioned. In Germany, too, younger doctors only know this active ingredient as a tool in researching the functions of the sodium pump. I have published a number of scientific articles on ouabain with the aim of correcting this deficit:

Ouabain - the insulin of the heart.
Int J Clin Pract. 2010 Nov;64(12):1591-4.

Rethinking heart failure.
Cardiol Res 2012;3(6):243-257

On the differences between ouabain and Digitalis glycosides.
Am J Ther. 2014 Jan-Feb;21(1):35-42.

Ouabain - the key to cardioprotection?
Am J Ther. 2014 Sep-Oct;21(5):395-402

"Why isn't clinical experience with ouabain more widely accepted?"
A J Physiol Heart Circ Physiol. 2014 Oct 15;307(8):H1262-3.

Ouabain and endogenous ouabain - Dr. Jekyll and Mr. Hyde of cardiac glycosides? British Journal of Medicine and Medical Research, 2015; 8(5): 477-484

Why Whip the Starving Horse When There Is Oats for the Starving Myocardium? Am J Ther. 2016 Sep-Oct;23(5):e1182-7.

Ouabain – a gift from paradise
Cardiovasc Disord Med, 2018; Volume 3(3): 1-2

In these papers the current and historical findings on the therapeutic efficacy and biochemical mechanisms of action of ouabain are described and discussed. Current research results confirm and explain the therapeutic experiences with ouabain. A clinical reassessment of this active substance is appropriate. The most concise results are described in brief in the following chapters. More detailed information and references can be found in the publications listed.

Ouabain and Coronary Heart Disease [12]

The properties of ouabain, its therapeutic effects, its molecular mechanisms of action, are based solely on its chemical structure. It is not influenced by scientific theories on the causes and course of diseases. Experimentally induced reduced blood flow to the heart muscle increases the acidity of the tissue and increases the lactate concentration in the blood. Increased acidity and lactate levels are also observed in angina pectoris patients. Ouabain reduces acidity and lactate levels in both reduced blood flow and angina pectoris. Myocardial theory and coronary theory offer different explanations. But all that counts is the effect observed on the patient. The therapeutic effects of ouabain cannot be deduced from hypotheses on the pathogenesis of angina pectoris or coronary heart disease.

Coronary heart disease is the most common cause of heart failure. With its acute manifestations, it is also the most frequent cause of death in the industrial nations. According to current teaching, coronary artery disease is caused by deposits in the walls of the coronary arteries. These lead to stiffening of the artery walls. It can reduce the cross-section of the vessel to a complete blockage. The blood circulation and, as a consequence, the oxygen supply to the heart muscles is reduced. There is a disproportion between oxygen demand and oxygen supply, which is called ischemia or coronary insufficiency. As the disease progresses, the probability of cardiac arrhythmia, heart attack and sudden cardiac death increases.

Coronary heart disease is a chronic disease that progresses over years to decades. Healing, in the sense of removing the deposits in the affected vessel walls, is not possible. By administering lipid-lowering

---

[12] Described in detail in: Ouabain - the key to cardioprotection? Am J Ther. 2014 Sep-Oct;21(5):395-402

drugs, statins, an attempt is made to slow the progression of the disease. In the advanced stage of the disease, heart failure, beta blockers, ACE inhibitors and diuretics are used.

Ernst Edens has achieved very good results in the treatment of angina pectoris, the leading symptom of coronary heart disease, with intravenous Strophanthin therapy. Sarre had similar effects with orally administered ouabain in the early 1950s. In coronary sclerosis with angina pectoris, Digitalis preparations increase the number of attacks, while ouabain reduces them [Sarre 1951, Sarre 1952]. Sarre concluded from his research *"Coronary insufficiency is the only indication where ouabain actually seems to be superior to other Digitalis drugs and even stands in some contrast to them"*.

As early as 1949, the physiologist Hermann Rein had shown in dogs that temporary ischemia (reduced blood flow) and hypoxia (oxygen deficiency in the blood with normal blood flow) triggered cardioprotective effects. He observed that ischemia as well as hypoxia apparently releases an active substance in the spleen which can be transferred from a donor animal to a recipient animal while maintaining the protective effect. Rein compared the effect of the body's own substance released by ischemia, which he called "Hypoxie-Lienin", with that of ouabain. He found a largely concurring effect. In contrast to Hypoxie-Lienin, however, ouabain has a longer lasting effect. Rein reports that after administration of ouabain *"the animal has simply become resistant to O_2 deficiency for hours"*.

Complex life forms such as mammals can only survive because they have sophisticated molecular defence and repair systems with which they protect their organisms. Because a constant, uninterrupted supply of oxygen is essential to sustain life, organisms possess innate defence mechanisms to increase tolerance to acute and chronic lack of oxygen. Many animal species that live in environments with variable oxygen supply exhibit a wide range of biochemical and physiological adaptations that allow them to withstand long periods of hypoxia. In many species, the immature heart possesses a higher resistance to oxygen deprivation than the mature heart. Human newborns exhibit a hypometabolic response to hypoxia, in common with other infant mammals. Populations residing at high altitude display lower incidences of hypertension and mortality rates for coronary heart disease and a reduced incidence of myocardial infarctions. Obviously, exposure to chronically reduced oxygen levels induces protection against these disease states. Data generated by animal studies strongly support the hypoxia-induced cardioprotection paradigm. A novel concept emerged from these data: exposure to moderate lack of oxygen triggers defence mechanisms to deal with reduced oxygen supply and induces endogenous cardio-protective programs. Intensive research on *"ischemic preconditioning"* - applying brief episodes of nonlethal ischemia and reperfusion to confer protection against a sustained episode of lethal ischemia and reperfusion injury - has shown that cardioprotection is indeed possible by conditioning of the heart with nonlethal ischemic episodes. The phenomenon of ischemic preconditioning is not only observed in cardiac tissue but occurs in other organs as well. Neuro-protective responses against stroke and injury of the brain and activation of intrinsic protective systems in patients undergoing liver surgery are well documented. Thus, it would seem that preconditioning represents a generalized adaptation to protect a wide variety of cells against stressful stimuli such as ischemia [Candilio 2013].

The protective mechanisms underlying ischemic conditioning are also activated by repeated interruption of blood supply by means of a blood pressure cuff in the arms (*remote preconditioning*). Remote preconditioning by ischemia in the arm releases one or more substances circulating in the blood that provide multiorgan protection [Kharbanda 2009]. As with *Hypoxie-Lienin* it possible to transfer the protective effect via blood transfer from a preconditioned donor to an unconditioned recipient. The structure of the active substance(s) is not yet known. (Although ouabain mimics the effects of *Hypoxie-Lienin*, there is no evidence that ouabain is identical with *Hypoxie-Lienin*. Its chemical structure is still unknown.) Encouraging experimental and clinical results are reported in the treatment of heart disease, stroke and Parkinson's disease. Many laboratories are working intensively to find low-molecular substances with which protective preconditioning can be induced (*pharmacological preconditioning*).

Stability in composition of the internal milieu of cells is maintained by transporting epithelia that exchange substances with the environment in a highly specific and regulated manner. Na/K-ATPase is a vital component of such exchange, because it not only transports Na+ and K+ vectorially, but it is secondarily responsible for the exchange of essential nutrients across epithelia. Hence, it has been suggested that ouabain may regulate the vectorial transport of Na+ across epithelia, accompanied by the downregulation of glucose, amino acids, ions, and other biologically relevant substances. This hypothesis underlines the general importance of ouabain for the regulation of the metabolism of cells.

Both animal and human findings indicate that reduced ATP utilization and, thus, metabolic downregulation is a key factor for "rapid" ischemic preconditioning in the heart. Ouabain has multiple effects on the cardiac metabolism that result in cardioprotection. Ischemia leads to a progressive accumulation of protons and lactic acid, ultimately inhibiting synthesis of adenosine triphosphate. Administration of ouabain in a myocardial infarct model in rats raises the pH of acidic cardiac tissue within a few minutes by up to 0.5 units. The pH sensitivity of the myocardium is well documented. A drop in the pH below 6.2 leads to irreversible damage. Therefore, in cardiac surgery, strict pH control is imperative. In the "Strophanthin Era" German surgeons routinely preconditioned the heart by applying 0.3 mg of ouabain preoperatively and thereby observed significantly fewer complications.

The molecular mechanisms underlying ischemic preconditioning are the subject of current research. There is evidence that the substances released in the organism during ischemia influence the activity of the sodium pump. The involvement of various signal cascades, which are also triggered by the interaction of ouabain with the sodium pump, has been proven. These include in particular the signalling cascades induced by protein kinase C and MAP kinase as well as glycogen synthase. Their functions are to open the calcium channels of the cell membrane, the mitochondria and the pores of the mitochondrial permeability transition. This results in better conservation of energy reserves. It is now considered certain that ouabain develops its cardioprotective effects by activating these ouabain-Na/K-ATPase signalosomes, which are independent of the ion pump function of the sodium pump. The concurring effects of ouabain and ischemic preconditioning make ouabain the ideal drug for pharmacological preconditioning. The safety, tolerability and effect of ouabain have been proven through decades of clinical use.

Current research on ischemic preconditioning confirms and explains the effect of ouabain in the treatment of coronary heart disease. The signal cascades induced by ischemic preconditioning as well as by ouabain lead to the protection of almost all internal organs. This also explains the *extracardial* protective effect of ouabain in stroke and kidney development. The effect of the signalosomes on the mitochondria important for energy supply was confirmed and also explains the clinical experience with ouabain, in which a positive effect on the energy balance of the heart had been observed. While digoxin was known as a "whip for the starving horse" because of its strong inotropy, ouabain was characterized by clinicians as "oats for the starving heart".

Ouabain and the energy balance of the heart[13]

A large number of clinical studies and experimental research results show that there is no demonstrable correlation between arteriosclerotic blood circulation disorders and heart failure [Marzilli 2012]. Many patients with angina pectoris and signs of ischemia have no detectable coronary arteriosclerosis and conversely, many patients with severe coronary arteriosclerosis have no chest pain and no evidence of myocardial ischemia. Extreme cases have been documented in which, despite complete occlusion of all three major coronary arteries, sufficient blood circulation in the heart and normal heart functions have been observed [Seiler 2009]. A distinct network of anastomoses and collaterals ensures sufficient blood flow to the heart muscle. Today we know that the failing heart is a unique example of a well-oxygenated heart in which a chronic mismatch between ATP synthesis and degradation results in loss of energy [Ingwall 2004].

The cholesterol hypothesis is crumbling. Today, cholesterol levels are differentiated according to HDL, *good* cholesterol and LDL, *bad* cholesterol. So far, all attempts to increase the level of good HDL have proved a failure. Roche's active ingredient dalcetrapib and Pfizer's torcetrapib have failed in major registration studies. In October 2015, Eli Lilly also discontinued a clinical trial involving 12,000 patients with the active substance evacetrapib.

Also, the invasive procedures of coronary revascularization (stents) and bypass of stenosis with high relapse rates have only minor effects on the survival rate of heart failure patients. The presence or absence

---

[13] Described in detail in: Rethinking heart failure. Cardiol Res 2012;3(6):243-257

of coronary arteriosclerosis is therefore of limited importance for the diagnosis and treatment of heart failure.

The heart is the motor of the body. It stimulates the circulation and distributes vital nutrients through the bloodstream and enables the exchange of substances and information between the various organs. Every day the heart beats over 100,000 times and pumps about 10 tons of blood through the body. In contrast to the skeletal muscles, there are no resting phases for regeneration in the heart muscle. The heart cannot be controlled consciously. The heart performs exclusively by contractions of the heart muscle, whose strength and frequency are adjusted to the respective need. It regulates the pumping power via the contraction force, the beat frequency, the stroke volume and the size of the heart chambers (hypertrophy). This exceptionally efficient organ reacts very flexibly to changing requirements. The conveying capacity is very different. It varies between 0.3 ml per minute and gram of heart muscle at rest and 5 - 6 ml per minute and gram during physical exertion.

The heart has an enormous need for energy. This is covered by high rates of adenosine triphosphate (ATP) synthesis and hydrolysis. The ATP supply of the heart cell is completely converted within seconds. The heart processes approx. 6 kg ATP per day. Mitochondria are the center of energy production. These take up about 30% of the volume of a heart cell. An important substrate for the heart is oxygen. At a heart rate of 60 to 70 beats per minute, the oxygen consumption per gram of heart muscle is 20 times higher than that of a skeletal muscle at rest. The heart uses about 70-80% of the oxygen offered in the blood, compared to 30-40% in the skeletal muscles. Fats (60-80%) and glucose (20%) are the main energy substrates, small amounts of ketones (lactate) and amino acids are also metabolized. Protons are produced during both the production and consumption of ATP. On reaction with oxygen in the mitochondria these are converted into water.

The classical basic idea in ischemic heart diseases, that these are essentially due to a deficit in the oxygen supply to the heart, suggests that the heart is dependent on oxygen supply. However, studies have shown that the heart can survive not only minutes but hours and days with only limited oxygen supply. As early as 1966 Hochrein showed on guinea pigs heart-lung preparations that hearts can survive even in the complete absence of oxygen supply. Through infusion of glucose, insulin and potassium salts, hypoxic heart failure and respiratory arrest induced by nitrogen respiration could be remedied despite continuous nitrogen respiration [Hochrein 1966]. In 1992, Webster and his team reported that heart muscle cells remain viable and contractile for one week in vitro with no oxygen if glucose is continuously supplied and the extracellular pH is kept within the physiological range [Graham 2004]. These experiments show that oxygen deficiency does not necessarily lead to the death of heart muscle cells. Lack of energy and hyperacidity cause the death of the heart cells.

In order to remain viable under oxygen deficiency, the cells must be continuously supplied with glucose from which sufficient ATP can be produced via anaerobic glycolysis if required. In addition, it must be ensured that the resulting acid is removed. If these conditions are not fully met, acidosis causes cell death. Acidosis also causes the chest pain frequently observed in angina pectoris. Specific acid-sensitive ion channels trigger anginoid chest pain.

The autonomic nervous system regulates the activity of the heart. In patients with heart failure, vagus tone is reduced, while sympathetic tone is increased. Risk factors for cardiovascular diseases such as obesity, high blood pressure and smoking are all characterized by increased sympathetic activation. Increased sympathetic tone is also observed in depression, anxiety, social isolation and chronic stress. The degree of sympathetic activation is an important and independent determinant in the prognosis of myocardial and cerebral diseases. Catecholamines are the neurotransmitters of the sympathetic nervous system. In heart failure patients, increased plasma catecholamine levels correlate closely with increased mortality.

Even as early as the 1930s the German pharmacologist Hans Gremels identified some fundamental correlations between the neurotransmitters of the sympathetic nervous system, epinephrine, and the para-sympathetic nervous system, acetylcholine, on myocardial performance and metabolism [Gremels 1946]. Due to the surgical intervention, the heart in a heart-lung preparation is a failing heart. The lifetime of denervated dog heart-lung preparations can be multiplied by infusion of acetylcholine and epinephrine ("humoral innervation") with simultaneous increase of the efficiency of cardiac workload, indicating that the autonomous nervous system through release of its transmitters is essential for the activity of the heart. Gremels observed that the sympathetic stimulation increases oxygen consumption of the heart, while the parasympathetic activity decreases oxygen consumption. Catecholamines like epinephrine stimulate sympathicotonic dissimilation that is counterbalanced by vagotonic assimilation stimulated by acetylcholine. The vagotonic assimilation regulates the quiescent state of the organism. Through counter regulatory control it is triggered by sympathicotonic activity, which in addition determines its intensity. Gremels thus revealed dynamic interactions of sympathetic and parasympathetic nervous systems that today are known as "accentuated antagonism". Vagal "tone" predominates over sympathetic tone at rest. Under normal physiological conditions, parasympathetic stimulation will inhibit tonic sympathetic activation. Elevated sympathetic tone is overridden by intense vagus nerve discharge. Due to this "accentuated antagonism" the effects of catecholamines are very sensitive to changes in concentration. Whereas high concentrations induce increased oxygen consumption, lower concentrations show a decrease in oxygen consumption due to counter regulatory functional activation of the parasympathetic system.

Gremels interpreted increases in oxygen consumption as a consequence of impaired stimulation by acetylcholine and insulin on glucose utilization and glycogen synthesis, which results in a predominance of sympathetically induced oxygen-consuming metabolic activity. He classified such an increase in oxygen consumption as "energetic insufficiency". Energetic insufficiency always precedes depressed contractile function. Current experiments confirm this observation. Alterations in the myocardial creatine kinase system precede the development of contractile dysfunction in beta(1)-adrenergic receptor transgenic mice. Transgenic overexpression of myofibrillar isoform-creatine kinase in the failing heart of mice significantly increases the rate of in vivo ATP delivery that induces enhanced systolic function, and improves survival. Data from the Studies of Left Ventricular Dysfunction indicate that neurohumoral excitation actually precedes the clinical onset of heart failure. Nevertheless, it still is a widespread assumption that neuro-endocrine activation and its consequences for myocardial metabolism is a reaction to changes in hemodynamics. In a recent scientific position statement from the Translational Research Committee of the Heart Failure Association of the European Society of Cardiology it is asserted:

"Complex autonomic nervous system imbalances exist in chronic heart failure. These can be simplified as excessive sympathetic nervous system activation and withdrawal of parasympathetic nervous system activity. These changes may initially be considered as short-term compensatory responses to the haemodynamic alterations that result from abnormal cardiac function." [van Bilsen 2017].

The experimental and clinical evidence already referred to clearly suggests that autonomic dysregulation and subsequent changes in myocardial metabolism precede heart failure. This is in accordance with the basic laws of physics: any change in contractile output requires preceding provision of energy. First you step on the gas, then the engine accelerates, when you step down from the gas pedal, the engine then slows down, not vice versa.

In Gremels' dog heart-lung preparations acetylcholine-mediated absorption of glucose from the blood always preceded reduction in oxygen consumption, which was then followed by increase in contractile output. Acetylcholine enhanced the effects of insulin. Addition of glucose, too, increased the effects of acetylcholine, presumably through the stimulation of insulin release. Addition of cardiotonic steroids yielded comparable effects. Therapeutic concentrations of Strophanthus- and Digitalis-glycosides multiplied the effect of acetylcholine dramatically by a factor of 1,000. Just like acetylcholine the

glycosides first corrected the impaired sugar assimilation, then reduced increased oxygen consumption and finally improved the cardiac
output back to normal.

As early as the 1930s, several researchers (Gollwitz-Meier, Gremels,
and others) had shown that when analysing ischemic conditions of the
heart muscle, not only the ratio of oxygen supply and demand in the
myocardium, but also the *oxygen consumption* of the heart controlled
by the vegetative nervous system should be taken into account. In the
1950s and 1960s, Raab, Selye, Schimmert and many other scientists
proved beyond doubt that excessive sympathetic activity caused an
extreme increase in the heart's oxygen consumption, which led to
oxygen deficiency and necrosis (death of heart cells). They have also
shown that not only physical *stress* but also emotional excitement
(emotional stress) leads to increased release of stress hormones (adrenaline, noradrenaline, cortisol) and thus to increased oxygen demand
of the heart. Recent studies show that a high percentage of all angina
pectoris attacks and heart attacks are triggered by emotional stress.

Excessive sympathetic activity due to the release of excessive
amounts of catecholamine leads to heart damage. In low concentrations, catecholamines have beneficial effects on cardiac function (including positive inotropic effects). High concentrations of catecholamines, on the other hand, damage the heart under chronic exposure.
They increase oxygen demand and accelerate aerobic glycolysis,
which leads to excess protons. They stimulate the lipolysis of trigly-
cerides and thus release fatty acids and other protons. Serum concentrations of norepinephrine correlate closely with the degree of disease
and a poor prognosis in heart failure. Catecholamines interfere with
oxidative phosphorylation in the mitochondria. In sum, excessive
sympathetic tone via high catecholamine concentrations leads to the
accumulation of protons and thus to acidosis-induced cell death.

If the proton concentrations in the heart muscle cell cannot be regulated by oxidative phosphorylation in the mitochondria, an alternative
mechanism of proton utilization takes effect. Pyruvate (pyruvic acid)
is reduced to lactate (lactic acid) by consuming protons. The formati-

on of lactate (lactic acid) is therefore not the cause of acidosis ("lactate acidosis"), as is still wrongly asserted in textbooks. The reduction
of pyruvate to lactate consumes protons. Lactate formation is a protective measure of the cell against excessive acid production. Lactate
(lactic acid) is an indication of acidosis, but not a cause of acidosis
[Robergs 2004]. In heart failure patients, the lactate level in the blood
is elevated.

Today we know that in heart failure - independent of its pathogenesis
– there always is a disturbance of the myocardial metabolism [Ingwall
2009]. There is no lack of oxygen. The utilization of nutrients is disturbed. That is why Heinrich Taegtmeyer asked the famous and still
unanswered question *"Why does the heart fail in the midst of plenty?"*
[Taegtmeyer 2002]. The capacity of mitochondria, the cell's power
plant, for the oxidation of sugar and fats is reduced. The risk of heart
disease increases with age. Older patients have an almost 50% lower
oxidative capacity of mitochondria. The extent of the impairment in
energy supply correlates with the observed mortality. Obviously it is
not a limited availability of nutrients or oxygen, but the ability to process the available substrates and oxygen, which leads to heart failure,
disturbed by predominance of sympathetic tone. Here ouabain inter-
venes to protect. Particularly weak hearts ("old age heart") often react
very positively to ouabain. That is why Ernst Edens called ouabain
milk of old age.

If the aerobic - oxygen-based - metabolism fails, the energy deficit of
the heart can only be compensated by anaerobic metabolism - without
oxygen. As long as the energy provided by anaerobic metabolism
keeps the blood flow at a sufficient level, excess protons are washed
out and acidosis-induced infarction is prevented.

Ouabain modulates the metabolism of the heart cell. Fraenkel and
Edens had already pointed out that Strophanthin influences the metabolism. A synergistic effect with insulin was already known at that
time. In low concentrations, insulin increases ouabain exposure and
reduces toxicity. This effect has also been used in practice. Ouabain
solutions were diluted with dextrose solution before injection. This

not only prevented excessive peak concentrations with too rapid injection as protection against the dreaded Strophanthin death. At the same time, dextrose induces the release of insulin and thus increases the effect of ouabain.

In heart failure patients, lactate levels in the blood are elevated and can be lowered by administering ouabain. Ouabain enhances the metabolic effect of acetylcholine (the neurotransmitter of the parasympathetic nervous system) and inhibits an increased oxygen consumption induced by adrenalin. It promotes fatty acid metabolism, stimulates glycogen synthesis and increases protein synthesis in the heart muscle. In animal experiments, ouabain increases the ratio of acetyl coenzyme A to coenzyme A in the myocardium, which indicates an activation of the metabolism. Hermann Rein has shown in dogs on ligation of the coronary arteries the animals have become "resistant to O_2 deficiency for hours" after ouabain administration. In a myocardial infarction induced by ligation in rat and rabbit hearts, the pH value in the heart muscle tissue decreases significantly. Administration of ouabain increases the pH value of the acidic heart tissue within a few minutes by up to 0.5 pH units.

The metabolic effect of ouabain proves a pronounced effect on the autonomic nervous system. Stimulation of the parasympathetic system and inhibition of the sympathetic system are indicated by the promotion of energy supply while at the same time inhibiting excessive energy consumption. The neurotransmitter of the parasympathetic nervous system is acetylcholine. In small doses, ouabain releases acetylcholine and increases its concentration in the heart. It activates parasympathetic influence. In his double-blind study with k-Strophanthin and digoxin in heart patients, Agostini observed that k-Strophanthin reduces catecholamine levels in the serum of patients [Agostini 1994]. It inhibits the sympathetic nervous system.

With this active profile, ouabain is the ideal remedy for the treatment of heart failure. Activity and metabolism of the heart are controlled by the vegetative nervous system. Its antagonistic components - sympathetic nervous system and parasympathetic nervous system - interact with each other in a specific way. Stimulation or inhibition of one always causes a partial stimulation/inhibition of the opponent. This interaction is called *accentuated antagonism*. Modulation of the vegetative nervous system that affects both components will therefore always be more effective than the mere blocking of receptors of a component as practiced in therapy with beta blockers and ACE inhibitors.

Ouabain and Digitalis[14]

In the 19th century, Schmiedeberg founded the dogma, which is still valid today, that all cardiac-active glycosides have the same qualitative effects. According to current doctrine, there are only minor quantitative differences. Differences in effect were also denied in the protocol to the Heidelberg Tribunal: "Different effects of Strophanthin and other cardiac glycosides on the musculature of the left and right ventricle have not been proven." This assessment is supported by the observation that in sufficiently high concentrations all cardiac glycosides bind to the sodium pump and inhibit its activity. Inhibition of the sodium pump brings many physiological processes to a standstill. Inhibition of the sodium pump leads to immediate cardiac death. It explains the toxic effect of cardiac glycosides! This puts Fraenkel's question, *"Are we at all entitled to conclude from the toxic effect of a Digitalis body on the frog's heart on its therapeutic effect on humans?"* on a new, molecularly based foundation.

Ernst Edens and Albert Fraenkel denied this question on the basis of their clinical observations. In the Strophoral dispute in the 1950s, changes in the ECG (ST changes) were required to demonstrate an effect of orally administered Strophanthin. Today we know that the ST changes in the ECG are signs of ischemic conditions, as they also occur in patients suffering from angina pectoris. These characteristic changes in the ECG are also observed after Digitalis treatment. In stress tests of healthy persons patients taking Digitalis, glycoside-induced ST alterations occur in 30-40% of the test persons. Therefore,

---

[14] detailed in: On the differences between ouabain and digitalis glycosides.
Am J Ther. 2014 Jan-Feb;21(1):35-42.
Ouabain and endogenous ouabain - Dr. Jekyll and Mr. Hyde of cardiac glycosides?
British Journal of Medicine and Medical Research, 2015; 8(5): 477-484
Why Whip the Starving Horse When There Is Oats for the Starving Myocardium?
Am J Ther. 2016 Sep-Oct;23(5):e1182-7.

Digitalis preparations must be discontinued in time before measuring a stress ECG (1 week break for digoxin, 3 weeks break for digitoxin). Also with the changes in the ECG one had tried to conclude from the toxic effect on the therapeutic effect. The situation is no different with the inhibition of the sodium pump. It is the common characteristic of all cardiac glycosides for toxicity. It is not possible to derive their therapeutic effect from total inhibition of the sodium pump. As a way out, therefore, the hypothesis that the therapeutic effect of glycosides is based on only *partial inhibition* of the sodium pump has been put forward in all textbooks [15]. Through partial inhibition, more sodium remains in the cell and the intracellular and extracellular sodium concentration is equalized, the Na/Ca exchange is inhibited and the calcium concentration in the cell increases. The increased calcium concentration results in improved contractility.

This hypothesis has been repeatedly questioned by experimental investigations. The guiding effect of Digitalis is a pronounced inotropic effect. Okita has described the separation of inotropic and toxic effects in several studies [Okita 1977]. Lüllmann has shown that the inotropic effect does not correlate with the degree of inhibition of the sodium pump. However, there is a close correlation between electro-

---

[15] This hypothesis was put forward in 1969 by Morcedai Blaustein [Baker 1969]. He described in 2013 how he came to it: "I immediately recognized that NCX - Natrium-Calcium-Pumpe - must be widely distributed in both tissues and species, including vertebrate heart. Therefore, since NCX apparently functions in the heart, it is the missing link to the puzzle that had stumped me ever since my first studies on the Na+ pump and, as an intern, my use of digitalis to treat patients with heart failure: How does Na+ pump inhibition by cardiotonic steroids increase the force of contraction of the heart? Because of both my clinical and research experiences, I frequently thought about this enigma. Here was the answer: raising [Na+]i promotes net Ca2+ gain by NCX, and thereby enhances cardiac contraction. That 'Eureka! moment' was even more thrilling than the discovery of NCX itself. I was, for a brief time, the only one in the world who understood how cardiotonic steroids enhance cardiac contraction! I was so exhilarated that I went off, alone, to the nearby Green Lantern restaurant, for a fine celebratory dinner with a bottle of claret." [Blaustein 2013].

lyte composition and toxicity [Lüllmann 1982, 1984]. Liu has confirmed these results 20 years later [Liu 2000]. Wasserstrom reports that the strength of inotropy varies greatly with the structure of glycosides, while toxicity hardly varies with structural changes [Wasserstrom 1988, 1991]. A detailed discussion of the inotropic effects in relation to the inhibition of the sodium pump was published in 2005 [Wasserstrom 2005].

Compounds of different substance classes inhibit the sodium pump. However, none of these substances has a cardiac effect comparable to cardiac glycosides. Rats are quite insensitive to cardiac glycosides. The affinity of cardiac glycosides to the rat's sodium pump is significantly lower than that of other animals. The lethal dose of cardiac glycosides in rats is several orders of magnitude higher than that for sensitive animal species. When administered intraperitoneally, the lethal dose (LD50) of ouabain in mice is 1.2 mg/kg body weight, while the lethal dose in rats is 125 mg/kg. Orally administered LD50 of digoxin is 28.3 mg/kg in rats and 3.5 mg/kg in guinea pigs. The lethal dose for oral digitoxin is 56 mg/kg in rats and 0.2 mg/kg in cats. These findings also indicate that inhibition of the sodium pump is responsible for the toxicity but not for the therapeutic effect of cardiac glycosides.

For the experimental determination of the inhibitory effect of cardiac glycosides on the sodium pump, different methods have been used, which have led to very different results. Preparations of the sodium pump from both human and animal tissue were used. The measuring methods - medium, reagents, reaction time - were not standardised. A research group led by Alexei Bagrov and Amir Askari has determined the binding constants of several cardiac glycosides on purified enzyme preparations from human kidney tissue and from kidney tissue of pigs [Gable 2017]. Corresponding inhibitory effects of cardiac glycosides on Na/K-ATPases from human and pig kidney were measured. The inhibition constant (Ki value) of ouabain is 1.22 ± 0.09 µM, the Ki value of digoxin was determined to 3.2 ± 0.22 µM. In contrast, the therapeutic concentrations in the treatment of heart disease are < 0.5

nM for ouabain and 1 - 2 nM for digoxin. The concentrations of cardiac glycosides required to inhibit the sodium pump are thus 1,000 times higher than the concentrations used for therapeutic purposes. This refutes the hypothesis that the therapeutic effect of cardiac glycosides is based on inhibiting the sodium pump.

In vivo experiments with mice have shown that the protective effect of ouabain in heart failure is not based on inhibition of the sodium pump, but is induced by activation of a specific kinase (phosphoinositide 3-kinase-α) [Wu 2015]. The authors conclude from their experiments: *"In conjunction with a wealth of available information on the clinical use of Digitalis drugs in man, the present findings also suggest the need for further studies on the potential use of these drugs for the prevention of heart failure as advocated nearly a century ago."*

The equation of inhibition of the sodium pump with therapeutic effect was formulated correctly at first as a hypothesis[16] but then mutated into a statement of facts after repeated, thoughtless repetition, omitting more and more details. This effect is often observed in science (lactate acidosis!). In medicine too, as in many other areas of life, the following applies freely in reference to George Orwell's "1984": "If everyone believes in the lie, the lie becomes the truth".

For ouabain, differences to Digitalis drugs are not only documented in clinical findings. There are also a number of clear differences at the

---

[16] The original text from 1969 is: "The observation that raising the internal sodium concentration increases calcium influx may help to explain the cardiotonic action of cardiac glycosides. Ouabain seems to have no direct effect on calcium movements, but it inhibits the Na-K pump in therapeutic doses and might increase the internal sodium concentration. If heart muscle behaves like squid nerve, a rise in internal sodium should promote calcium influx and increase the internal calcium concentration. Since muscle is probably activated by a release of calcium from the sarcoplasmic vesicles, or by entry of calcium from outside, an increase in the background level of calcium might improve the effectiveness of the action potential in turning on the contractile mechanism." [Baker 1969].

molecular level. Differences in pharmacokinetics are striking. The effect of ouabain starts very quickly within minutes, with digitoxin the full effect is only achieved after hours. This difference may be due to the fact that ouabain and Digitalis develop their effects in different cell compartments. Ouabain binds to the extracellular side of the cell membrane, digoxin and digitoxin enter the cell and bind to the intracellular ryanodine receptor. The lipophilic (fat-soluble) Digitalis glycosides are able to form cation-selective channels for calcium ions in lipid bilayers in cell cultures. The hydrophilic (water-soluble) ouabain is not able to do this. As described in previous chapters ouabain promotes the vagomimetic energy supply of the myocardium. Digitalis in many cases has the opposite effect. It sympathomimetically increases energy consumption, increases lactate concentration, lowers pH, and reduces protein synthesis.

The metabolic effects of cardiac glycosides illustrate their effect on the autonomic nervous system. Indeed, a table of the therapeutic and toxic effects of cardiac glycosides shows striking similarities to a tabulation of the combined effects of acetylcholine and adrenaline, the neurotransmitters of the autonomic nervous system [Runge 1975, 1977]. Lipophilic cardiac glycosides show increased sympathomimetic effects, hydrophilic cardiac glycosides such as ouabain show pronounced vagomimetic effects. Digoxin as a strong inotrope shows only weak effects on the autonomic nervous system. In Strophanthus derivatives, the modulation of the autonomic nervous system dominates a weak inotropic effect.

All cardiac glycosides show a pronounced dose-response relationship, often characterized by opposite effects at high versus low concentrations. Cardiac glycosides are prototypical examples of hormetic substances. In high concentrations they inhibit the sodium pump, in therapeutic concentrations Digitalis and ouabain stimulate the sodium pump [Godfraind 1986]. While low doses of Digitalis inhibit the sympathetic nervous system, high doses have been shown in animal experiments to stimulate the sympathetic system and cause cardiac arrhythmia [Gillis 1975]. In the cat's heart, low doses of ouabain inhibit spontaneous sympathetic activity in preganglionic sympathetic nerves. Higher doses of ouabain lead to an increase in sympathetic nerve activity and ventricular tachycardia [Gillis 1969]. Low concentrations of ouabain induce the proliferation (formation of new cells) of several cell types, while higher concentrations lead to apoptosis (programmed cell death).

Hormetric dose-response relationships are also observed in patients. Digoxin improves the neurohormonal profile in low doses in patients with heart failure. Dose increases have sympathomimetic effects [Newton 1996, Gheorghiade 1995]. Low doses of lanatoside C improve oxygen deficiency tolerance; high doses significantly reduce tolerance in angina pectoris patients [Sarre 1951, 1952]. K-Strophanthin (0.25 mg, IV application) and ouabain (3 mg, oral) improve oxygen deficiency tolerance in angina pectoris patients. The effects of the Digitalis derivative lanatoside C is pronounced dose dependent. 0.1 mg IV shows a slight improvement (but much less than the Strophanthus derivatives); 0.2 mg and 0.8 mg significantly reduce the oxygen deficiency tolerance. These experiments confirm the hormetic nature of cardiac glycosides. They show that the hormetic-dose-response curves of the glycosides, although basically similar, show considerable differences in concentration. Lanatoside C has only a limited dosage window in which it has a positive effect. Strophanthus derivatives offer a much wider therapeutic window. In clinical practice, the unique dose-response relationship of cardiac glycosides is of utmost importance.

All available scientific results of ouabain research leave no doubt that this active substance has a therapeutic and pharmacological profile which sets itself extremely positively apart from that of Digitalis glycosides. It is hoped that ouabain will soon be available again for the treatment of heart failure.

Ouabain protects the kidney and the brain

The therapeutic potential of ouabain is not limited to the treatment of heart disease. Similar to ischemic preconditioning, ouabain has the potential to protect other organs. Studies on animal models show that the kidneys are protected against malnutrition.

Chronic malnutrition with severe restrictions on protein intake is a serious socio-economic problem, especially in developing countries. Several scientific studies have shown a strong influence of reduced protein intake and other nutritional deficiencies on the development of cardiovascular and renal diseases. The consequences of malnutrition are particularly dramatic for embryos and young people. High blood pressure, heart disease and kidney disease are among the most common consequences of malnutrition. More than one billion people worldwide are affected.

Malnutrition-related diseases are not only a problem in developing countries. Extensive data collection on all births in Norway between 1967 and 2004 showed that low birth weight is associated with a 70% increased risk of kidney failure. Studies on autopsy material have confirmed that low birth weight is a sign of fetal growth restriction in humans. Low calorie intake in pregnant women, like placental insufficiency, leads to an irreversible loss of functional units of the kidney, the nephrons. Loss of nephrons is a major risk factor for chronic kidney disease and high blood pressure.

Cardiovascular and renal diseases are intertwined by hormonal mechanisms. Chronic kidney disease is associated with an increased risk of high blood pressure and cardiovascular disease. Chronic kidney disease is a major socio-economic burden in developed and developing countries. There are more than 20 million Americans who have signs of chronic kidney disease and are at risk of dying of kidney failure. The annual cost of treating kidney disease in the United States accounts for more than a quarter of Medicare spending. However, despite overwhelming evidence that foetal malnutrition endangers kidney development and leads to irreversible loss of nephrons and an increased risk of kidney disease and hypertension in later life, there is as yet no drug to alleviate the effects of malnutrition on foetal nephron formation.

A rersearch group led by Anita Aperia at the renowned Karolinska Institute in Stockholm has demonstrated in vivo in the rat model that ouabain prevents misdevelopments of the embryonic kidney caused by malnutrition [Li 2010]. Pregnant rats were on a low-protein diet and treated with low-dose ouabain (serum concentration of 1 ng/ml). In contrast to untreated animalso no adverse effects of malnutrition were observed in animals exposed to ouabain.

Mechanistic studies have shown that the protective effect of ouabain is triggered by activation of the Na/K-ATPase-IP3R signalosome [Khodus 2011]. When ouabain acts on the sodium pump in low nanomolar concentrations that do not affect the ion-pump function, the inositol 1,4,5-trisphosphate receptor (IP3R) is activated via protein-protein interaction. This generates oscillating intracellular calcium ion concentrations which activate the pleiotropic transcription factor nuclear factor kappa B (NF-kB). This calcium-dependent NF-kB activation protects against apoptosis and increases cell proliferation.

A group of Brazilian scientists from the Federal University of Rio de Janeiro has also been able to show in rats that protein kinase-induced signalling pathways are severely impaired by malnutrition, especially those of protein kinases A and C [Silva 2014]. Angiotensin receptors and activation of the MAPK/ERK1/2 signalling cascade are also involved. The MAPK/ERK1/2 signalling pathways seem to be of decisive importance for the regulation of physiological and pathological events. It is known that the MAPK/ERK1/2 signalling cascade can be influenced by interaction of ouabain with the sodium pump.

Autosomal dominant polycystic kidney disease (ADPKD) is an inherited disorder that occurs in 1:400-1:1,000 individuals worldwide.

The main manifestations of ADPKD appear in the kidney, with the formation of numerous epithelial-lined cysts that develop throughout the nephron and predominantly in collecting duct cells. Cysts progressively expand, impair renal function, and lead to end stage renal disease in 50% of the affected individuals by age 60. Many patients with ADPKD require dialysis or undergo transplant therapy. Finding therapeutic approaches to treat ADPKD is highly needed to relieve the physical burden of the patients that suffer from this disease as well as to decrease the health care costs associated with palliative measures used to prolong the life of these patients. Currently, there is no specific treatment for ADPKD approved in the United States. Identification of factors that favor cyst progression provides opportunities to halt or control cyst formation and the advancement and morbidity of the disease. The development of potential pharmacological approaches for ADPKD treatment has been directed toward interfering with the intracellular pathways governing cyst growth. New findings have identified ouabain as an important pro-cystogenic factor in ADPKD. Ouabain promotes the cystic characteristics of ADPKD cells [Venugopal 2017].

Activation of multiple signal transduction pathways by ouabain is not restricted to myocardial and kidney cells. By interaction with Na/K-ATPase in the brain, ouabain influences signal pathways that are well-known molecular targets of mood stabilizers and antipsychotics. Several studies suggest that ouabain-induced effects in the brain are involved in behavioral changes that mimic the phenotypes of bipolar disorder. Intracerebroventricular injection induces behavioral changes in rats resembling the manic phenotypes. An ouabain model for bipolar illness is the only available animal model that fulfils all essential criteria for an adequate animal model for this disease. These results conform with clinical experiences that indicate anxiolytic effects of ouabain. Heart patients report an improved mood, general freshness, and willingness to increased activity after ingestion of ouabain. In patients with endogenous depression, treatment with ouabain diminished the depth of depression. In this context, it is of interest that ouabain has been used with good results in clinical treatment of de-

mentia. In patients with the syndrome of cerebral malnutrition, ouabain therapy has proven very effective (positive nutrition effect)[17].
Such effects have not been observed with Digitalis glycosides.

These examples also prove the enormous gain in knowledge that research on Na/K-ATPase signalosomes has produced in recent years.
All these new findings highlight the untapped therapeutic potential of
ouabain.

---

[17] Complete list of references for the mentioned effects of ouabain on the brain is available in:
Fürstenwerth H, On the differences between ouabain and Digitalis glycosides. Am J Ther. 2014
Jan-Feb;21(1):35-42.

Paradigm shift in pharmaceutical research

The Medicines Act had many effects on the process of developing new drugs. Drug safety for the protection of patients has been greatly improved. However, the far-reaching structural change in the pharmaceutical industry induced by the Medicines Act is hardly noticed. Only large, financially strong companies can still take the risk of developing new drugs. Small and medium-sized enterprises do not have the necessary resources. The influence of the many institutions involved in the development of a new drug has also shifted dramatically. Until the 1960s, the influence of university clinicians was extremely important. Companies made new preparations available to them for testing. In consultation with the companies, the clinicians were free to decide how and at which patient pool they carried out their trials and assessments. The clinicians' verdict often decided whether a drug was offered for sale. Standard procedures have been prescribed by the Medicines Act. It needs to be agreed with the regulatory authorities which studies are to be carried out and how. Since then, the university hospital has only been a service provider for the pharmaceutical industry. Clinical studies are still conducted at university institutes on behalf of the companies. However, the companies alone decide which drug candidates are included in clinical development and in which indication they are tested. If there are positive results in the prescribed studies, the decision to launch a certain drug on the market is made solely by the companies. The proof of safety and efficacy of a new drug required by the Medicines Act is provided by industrial companies alone. The companies have a defacto monopoly on the supply of new medicines. They use the clinical trials to determine which drugs become guidelines based treatments.

A flood of new scientific knowledge has revolutionized the process of developing new drugs. Today, the search for new active substances is almost exclusively based on an understanding of the biochemical basis of diseases. In pharmaceutical research, the receptor- or mechanism-based approach dominates.

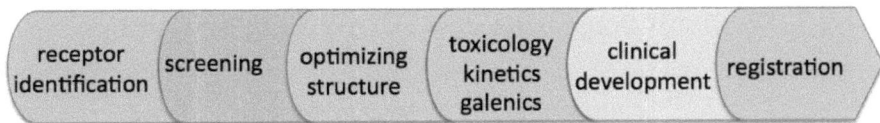

receptor identification → screening → optimizing structure → toxicology kinetics galenics → clinical development → registration

In the first step in the search for a new drug, molecular receptors are identified which are assumed to play an essential role in the development of diseases. These hypothetical drug targets are verified in animal models. If it can be shown in the animal model that the addressed receptors are disease-relevant, substances that affect these enzymes are tested in multi-stage iterative procedures. The identified key substances ("hits") are further refined. Finally, selected compounds are subjected to extensive toxicological and pharmacological tests in the laboratory and on animals. Only substances with an advantageous profile enter clinical development. This runs in three phases. In Phase I, tolerability and safety are tested on healthy volunteers. In phase II, the first efficacy data and the optimal dosage of the drug are determined on sick patients. In phase III, all efficacy and safety data required for approval are determined in large-scale clinical studies.

Only clinical studies show whether the selected molecular receptors are really disease-relevant and whether the safety data found in the animal model also apply to humans. The success rates are frustratingly low. Less than ten percent of drug candidates entering very cost-intensive clinical development reach the market.

All data determined for an active substance in development are transferred to a comprehensive approval dossier. All data on pharmaceutical quality (production, testing, shelf life), preclinical testing and the three clinical trial phases are documented and evaluated. This dossier is submitted to the regulatory authorities and serves as a basis for deciding whether the medicinal product is to be authorised. The entire process - from the beginning of receptor identification to registration - extends over a period of more than ten years.

The Truly Staggering Cost Of Inventing New Drugs

Research Spending Per New Drug 1997-2011		
Company	Number of dugs approved	R&D Spending per drug ($Mil)
AstraZeneca	5	11,790.93
GlaxoSmithKline	10	8,170.81
Sanofi	8	7,909.26
Roche Holding AG	11	7,803.77
Pfizer Inc.	14	7,727.03
Johnson & Johnson	15	5,885.65
Eli Lilly & Co.	11	4,577.04
Abbott Laboratories	8	4,496.21
Merck & Co Inc	16	4,209.99
Bristol-Myers Squibb Co.	11	4,152.26
Novartis AG	21	3,983.13
Amgen Inc.	9	3,692.14

Sources: InnoThink Center For Research In Biomedical Innovation; Thomson Reuters Fundamentals via FactSet Research Systems

The research and development of new drugs is a time-consuming and costly process. Due to the high failure rates, the costs of which are added to the cost of development for successful products, the expenditure required for the successful development of a new drug is already several billion dollars. For this reason, all research-based pharmaceutical and biotechnology companies are striving to systematically reduce the failure rate of their development products.

The simplest and most frequently used method is to only process active substances for receptors that have already been validated by commercial products and whose disease relevance is therefore known. This significantly reduces the failure rate in capital-intensive clinical trials. However, no real progress can be made with this strategy. Only known classes of active ingredients are optimized. Activity profiles are gradually improved. This results in fake innovations. Hence the old saying applies: "If you always do what you've always done, you always get what you've always gotten."

The quality of new drugs is therefore increasingly doubted. A study carried out on behalf of the Techniker Krankenkasse (a health insurance company) concludes that new drugs are often not associated with any discernible therapeutic progress and therefore do not represent any real therapeutic innovations, but in many cases only have to be addressed as "commercial innovations" whose use makes therapies more expensive without offering patient-relevant additional benefits [Windt 2013]. Further studies confirm this assessment.

A study published in *Health Affairs* shows that the effectiveness of new drugs has declined sharply since the 1970s compared to placebo [Olfson 2013]. The study included 315 clinical studies published in four of the leading medical journals (British Medical Journal, Journal of the American Medical Association, Lancet and New England Journal of Medicine) from 1966 - 2010 comparing a drug with a placebo. In the 1970s, new drugs were on average 4.5 times more effective than placebo. In the 1980s new drugs were less than four times better, in the 1990s only twice as good, and in the 2000s only 36 percent better than a placebo. The health magazine *Prescrire* already rated only 17 of the 984 new drugs approved in the US since 2001 as "real progress" in 2011 [Prescrire 2011]. *Nature Reviews Drug Discovery* has published a survey of 184 specialists, according to which doctors prefer older drugs to new ones as "transformative" [Kesselheim 2013].

The marginal effects of new drugs are concealed by showing the effects determined in the clinical studies not in absolute but in relative values. With the controversial statins administered to reduce cholesterol levels, the absolute effect is about one percent, i.e. out of 100 patients treated, only in one a heart attack is prevented. However, the relative effect is stated, which is often 30 to 50%.

The JUPITER study sponsored by AstraZeneca, which included 17,802 patients, showed a 54% relative reduction in heart attacks. The absolute effect in reduction of coronary events was less than one percentage point.

In Pfizer's ASCOT-LLA study with Lipitor (atorvastatin), heart attacks and deaths occurred in 3% of the placebo-treated control group compared to 1.9% in the Lipitor group. The improvement with Lipitor treatment was therefore only 1.1 percentage points. In the official presentation of the results, however, reference was made to a 36 percent reduction in the risk of a heart attack.

Against this background, it is not surprising that stricter approval criteria are demanded worldwide to ensure that only genuine therapeutic innovations with significantly better efficacy are approved instead of pseudoinnovations with only marginal advantages for patients.

The mechanism based drug discovery that today is used almost exclusively in pharmaceutical research has a fundamental problem. It implies the premise that diseases are caused monocausally by malfunction of a receptor. A drug acts on this one receptor and thus leads to a causal correction of the disease pattern. However, only externally inflicted damage to the organism is caused monocausally: injuries, poisoning and infections. Diseases in the narrower sense, especially chronic diseases, are usually caused pluricausally. Chronic diseases develop slowly and often only show clear symptoms after years. This also applies to heart attack. It does not occur suddenly. Every heart attack is announced weeks, months or even years in advance. Initial symptoms are often ignored by the doctor and the patient. Several risk factors are nowadays associated with heart attack:

- Smoking,

- Stress,

- Blood pressure,

- Diabetes

- Coronary sclerosis,

- Overweight,

- Physical inactivity and

- Psychological factors

The interaction of several risk factors leads to the disease. Only when the endogenous protective mechanisms of the body, controlled by manifold feedback, collapse, *one* factor can manifest the disease. The final triggering factor, however, is not the only one that causes the barrel to overflow. An active substance found with the mechanism-based research approach only addresses one risk factor at a time and thus inevitably has only a minor effect on the complexity of the underlying disease. However, every therapy requires a comprehensive approach. This aspect has not yet been sufficiently taken into account in pharmaceutical research.

Medicine and Science

Today, medicine is based on scientific principles. This also applies to the development and testing of new drugs. The clinical studies carried out as part of the approval of a new drug suggest that the efficacy and harmlessness of a drug have been scientifically proven. This assumption is only partially true. In a strict interpretation of scientific principles, there can be no positive proof of the efficacy of a drug. The philosopher Karl Popper pointed out that there is no positive proof in science [Popper 1935]. Hypotheses are not proven, they are only considered true until refuted. The scientific approach to support a hypothesis is to try to falsify it. If the hypothesis cannot be refuted, it is considered true. From a scientific point of view, a clinical study to prove efficacy should therefore aim to refute the hypothesis of efficacy. Accordingly, the studies should be planned and carried out. In practice, however, approval studies are designed by the pharmaceutical companies in such a way that it is highly unlikely that negative results will result, i.e. that the hypothesis of efficacy is not falsified. The scientifically correct question would be: How must a study be designed to show that the drug has no effect? Common practice asks: How must a study be designed in order to exclude ineffectiveness? Patients and narrow indications are selected accordingly. One illustrative example is the heart failure drug Entresto® (active ingredient: valsartan/sacubitrile combination) from Novartis, which was approved in summer 2015. In a clinical trial involving 8,442 patients (PARADIGM-HF), advantages over standard medication with an ACE inhibitor (enalapril) were observed. Of patients treated with Entresto® for three years, 6.7 percent died less than those treated with enalapril (21.8 versus 28.5 percent). However, nine percent more angioedema (itchy swelling of the skin and mucous membranes) was recorded with Entresto® compared to enalapril (19 versus 10 percent). The cardiological organizations celebrate Entresto® as a paradigm shift in the treatment of heart failure. In the assessments by cardiological experts, the patients were preselected in the PARADIGM-HF study. In a phase of the study known in the industry as "wash-out" or "roll-in", all patients who showed signs of intolerance or no positive effects were excluded. Of 10,521 patients, 2,079 were rejected and only 8,442 were included in the evaluation of the study [Medscape 2014, NEJM 2014]. Such studies do not meet scientific standards. In the medical practice, studies designed in this way lead to the fact that the doctor can only prescribe Entresto® on suspicion. There is no "wash-out" preselection for him. What practical benefits for the medical practice do studies such as PARADIGM-HF have? What criteria should general practitioners use to select patients for treatment with Entresto®? As in pre-scientific times, patients become test subjects.

The diversity of new technologies and research methods, especially the decoding of the human genome, has profoundly changed our understanding of diseases and their causes. Today, diseases are often only defined on the basis of molecular, biochemical parameters. Parameters mutate into diseases. Medicines are authorised if they alter biochemical parameters without proof of a cure or prolongation of life. High cholesterol levels (LDL) are considered a disease, even if patients do not show any symptoms. Active substances from the class of PCSK9 inhibitors for lowering LDL values were approved in Europe and America in summer 2015 without proof of therapeutic benefit and may now be advertised and used as a means of preventing heart diseases. Amgen, manufacturer of the PCSK9 inhibitor Repatha® states: "The effect of Repatha on cardiovascular morbidity and mortality has not yet been determined." [Amgen 2015].

A reduction in LDL cholesterol was also the basis for the approval of the first statin in 1987, seven years before the Scandinavian Simvastatin Survival Trial was the first study to provide evidence of a clinical effect[18]. The pivotal studies of other statins also used a reduction in

---

[18] 100 patients need six years of Simvastatin treatment to avoid four fatal and seven non-fatal heart attacks.

LDL cholesterol as postulated evidence of positive effects in cardio-vascular diseases. Clinical studies as evidence of therapeutic effects were not available for the approval of statins.

Biochemical indicators become an end in themselves. The lower the guideline values for cholesterol, blood pressure or other parameters are set, the higher the number of people who are defined as *ill* and need medication. Research is abused for the generation of "diseases". With the lowering of the blood sugar limit from 110 milligrams per deciliter of blood (mg/dl) to 100 mg/dl in 2003, the number of diabetics in the USA rose from four to 30 million at one stroke. A year later, Europe also adopted this value. People without symptoms became diabetics (type 2) by measurement and require medication. In the USA, the lowering of cholesterol levels from 240 to 200 mg/dl had turned over 42 million people into patients. The reduction of high blood pressure from 160 to 90 mm Hg to the current 140/90 had resulted in an increase of 15 million patients.

The results of a study published in November 2015 (SPRINT) are now prompting cardiological organizations to recommend lowering the guideline value for blood pressure to 120 to 90 mm Hg [Sprint 2015]. In the study, patients whose blood pressure had been drug-adjusted to 120/90 mm Hg had a slightly lower mortality rate than patients whose blood pressure had been left at 140/90 mm Hg. In order to prevent a death over the study period of 3.26 years, 90 people had to be treated. To prevent cardiovascular death, 172 patients had to be treated for 3.26 years. At the same time, there was an increase in adverse events in the intensively treated group, including hypotension (plus 70%), syncope (circulatory collapse, plus 36%) and acute kidney damage or renal dysfunction (plus 64%). Nevertheless, Prof. Dr. Martin Hausberg, chairman of the German Hypertension League, is certain: "This study will have an impact on the guidelines worldwide - it is not yet clear exactly in what form - but it will undoubtedly have an impact." All leading German daily and weekly newspapers reported on the"new" guideline values for blood pressure immediately after the publication of the SPRINT study. Another millions of people are becoming patients who have to take lifelong medication to lower their blood pressure.

The self-conception of medicine has changed. Only what is measurable is valid. Subjective feeling of patients is no longer accepted as a criterion of illness. Prof. Wollheim had already stated in the Heidelberg Tribunal: *"Unfortunately, the subjective feeling of the patient is the worst guideline that we have for the assessment of any therapeutic procedure. We no longer live in the age of a purely revelatory medicine, but of a science-based medicine. As doctors, we must be committed to science. Otherwise we're healers."* With such a self-image of medicine, it comes as no surprise that more and more patients are seeking refuge with providers of alternative healing methods and often fall into the network of obscure sects.

Diseases traditionally manifest themselves in symptoms that the patient perceives. From the symptoms observed the physician can draw conclusions about the type of disease and recommend an adequate therapy and prescribe suitable medication. Chronic diseases are usually not caused monocausally, but result from the interaction of several factors, which are nowadays referred to as *risk factors.* The concept of risk factors has its origin in the Framingham study.

In the USA, as in many other countries, it had been observed in the 1940s that cardiovascular diseases had skyrocketed and had become the most frequent cause of death. The United States Public Health Service therefore initiated a study in 1948 to find out what factors caused the increase in diseases such as heart attacks or strokes. A large-scale epidemiological survey has documented the habits and diseases of the inhabitants of Framingham, a small town near Boston in the US state of Massachusetts, for decades. First evaluations were published at the end of the 1950s. More than 1,000 papers on the results of the Framingham study have now been published. The Framingham study today is considered one of the most important epidemiological studies ever conducted.

The Framingham study identified three key parameters statistically associated with an increased risk of cardiovascular disease:

- high cholesterol levels

- high blood pressure

- high blood sugar levels

The common cause was identified as the "American way of life": a high-fat diet and a lack of exercise.

These findings led to large-scale public information campaigns in the 1960s to warn the population of the possible dangers of high cholesterol levels, high blood pressure and high blood sugar levels. Under the leadership of the National Institute of Health, a National High Blood Pressure Education Programme (NHBPEP) was established in 1972, in which numerous research organisations were involved. Since then, a Joint National Committee has regularly published recommendations for reducing and treating blood pressure that is considered too high. In 1985, the National Cholesterol Education Program (NCEP) was launched by the American Heart Association (AHA) to expand this campaign. This programme was also supported by numerous research organisations: American Heart Association, American Medical Association and American College of Cardiology. Since its foundation, NCEP has regularly issued recommendations for the treatment of patients with high cholesterol [19].

Blood pressure, cholesterol and blood sugar were branded as *risk factors*. With the catchphrase "know your numbers" the Americans were urged with massive publication campaigns to have their blood values checked regularly as a preventive measure and to adjust their lifestyle to increased values. These instructional programmes initially had little effect on the medical practice. This only changed when the pharmaceutical industry opened up possibilities to influence the values for

---

[19] In many countries, guidelines set by national expert committees apply. As a rule, these are based on American values.

blood pressure, cholesterol and blood sugar with suitable drugs [Greene 2007].

Initially, only patients with extreme blood pressure, cholesterol or blood sugar levels were treated with medication. Over the years, the values classified as in need of treatment have been steadily reduced. Today, the limits set in the treatment guidelines are so low that large parts of the population are classified as ill, regardless of whether they have symptoms or not. It is hardly possible to further reduce the limit values for cholesterol. An upper limit of 200 mg/dl has applied here since the mid-1980s. This means that 70 percent of the German population between the ages of 40 and 60 have a high cholesterol level. The average value for 40-year-old women in Austria is about 220 mg/dl, for men even 235 mg/dl. At the age of about 60 years, the sexes equalize at 245 mg/dl. Only towards the end of life does the value drop rapidly. It would therefore be much more rational to be afraid of a drop in cholesterol levels.

The differentiation between *healthy* and *sick is* no longer based on symptoms and complaints perceptible by doctors and patients. Regardless of a person's individual condition, statistical numerical values define who is classified as ill. Biochemical parameters are considered diseases that must be treated, even if the patient feels healthy and has no symptoms. Illness is no longer an individual condition. Disease is a statistical indicator.

The values which define blood pressure, cholesterol and blood sugar as pathological are negotiated by the corresponding medical specialist organisations. The basis are studies financed by pharmaceutical companies in which the effect of drugs on lowering blood values and on the influence of mortality is determined. All existing studies on the influence of drugs to reduce blood pressure, cholesterol and blood sugar on mortality show only marginal reductions in absolute mortality rates. The moral argument of acting as a precaution justifies the constant reduction in guide values and the massive use of drugs by patients without symptoms.

In his description of left-ventricle failure, Berthold Kern has identified symptoms and complaints that are characteristic of incipient heart failure. Ouabain can successfully treat these complaints, which can be noticed by doctors and patients. Even at the Heidelberg Tribunal in 1971, German university clinicians refused to acknowledge the symptoms described by Kern as symptoms of the disease. The patients treated by Kern were classified as healthy. A drug therapy is therefore not appropriate. The effect of ouabain could only be a placebo effect. Only symptoms of advanced heart failure (edema) were classified as requiring treatment. Today, the guidelines of the German medical societies go far beyond the early treatment of the initial symptoms of heart failure advocated by Fraenkel, Edens and Kern. The guidelines currently in force define asymptomatic biochemical indicators as diseases that need to be treated. The statistical risk for a probable disease is established as an independent clinical symptom. People defined as ill are prescribed drugs, although they have no subjective complaints. They cannot perceive the success of the therapy of their symptom-free disease. The determination of blood values alone indicates whether the drug treatment shows effects. It is to be hoped that medicine will again follow Ernst Eden's example and focus solely on the well-being of the patient. Patients should no longer be degraded to objects of commercial interest under the guise of science. Those who are serious about prevention should not prescribe lifelong therapy with drugs, some of which have considerable side effects[20]. For many patients, the diagnosis of being chronically ill despite the lack of symptoms represents a massive psychological burden. Psychosomatic complaints are the result. The quality of life decreases [Tijmstra 1990].

---

[20] In September 2012, the Federal Institute for Drugs and Medical Devices (BfArM) decreed that the expert information of all cholesterol-lowering drugs in the group of statins must point out the"risk of an increase in blood sugar levels and the development of a blood sugar disease (diabetes mellitus) as a possible class effect".

Drugs rightly occupy a central position in scientific medicine. However, the treatment should continue to focus on the sick patient as a unique and unmistakable personality. Drug treatment as part of a comprehensive therapy (change of lifestyle!) cannot be degenerated to correct biochemical indicators. Diseases are very often an integral part of a personal destiny that those affected have to deal with for life. This insight has been lost in todays handling of patients in the medical practice.

There is another context that has received little attention, which should lead us all to greater composure in dealing with diseases. If one presents the number of annual deaths per year in a population of people - e.g. the German population - as a logarithm, the resulting curve from the age of 10 to death shows an astonishing, straight-line dependence on age. The precondition is that all monocausal deaths due to environmental influences (injuries, poisoning, infections) are excluded from the statistics.

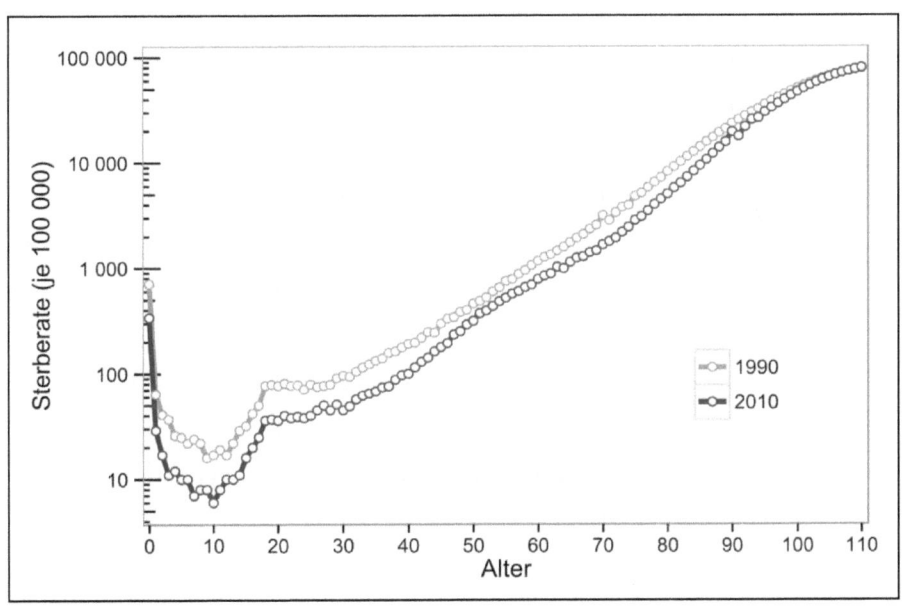

Mortality rate of the German population depending on age

This mortality line describes the probability of death in the German population as a whole. It documents a dominant influence of genes on life expectancy. Life expectancy is pretty much genetically determined [Schaefer 2000]. The gene pool determines how strong the endogenous defence and repair mechanisms of an organism are and how long it can defend itself against damaging influences. Drug treatments can only support the organism within the scope of the genetically determined possibilities. They cannot change the genetically determined limit. Illness and death are part of life. We should learn to deal calmly with this unalterable fact. Excessive use of medication cannot change this. But it reduces the quality of life.

Cornavita[21]

The incidence of heart failure is increasing. The prognosis of heart failure is still poor with mortality similar or even higher than with many common types of cancer, 5-year mortality being 56% for men and 45% for women. Using conventional treatments (Betablockers, angiotensin converting enzyme inhibitor, aldosterone antagonists) do not cure but alter the natural history of the disease. More patients are surviving to a stage of advanced chronic heart failure. There is an unmet need for better treatments. In the face of major disappointments following failure in large-scale clinical trials with two promising compounds (nesiritid and serelaxin [Cotter 2017]), several authors have expressed deep frustration about the state of research on heart failure [Packer 2018, Mebazaa 2018]. It is doubted that we have sufficient understanding of the course of the disease. As Milton Packer puts it: *"Our major need is not to propose novel therapies to be given only during the acute heart failure event, but instead, to develop new drugs to prevent these events by acting to change the course of the underlying disorder. Our current focus is obsessed with caring for the patient during hospitalization; instead, we need to ensure that the patient is managed well between hospitalizations. Such a change in strategy has major implications for our understanding of heart failure, the development of new drugs, and the goals of health delivery systems."* [Packer 2018].

But on a closer look these recent clinical failures do not come surprisingly. The drugs in question - nesiritid and serelaxin – are both vasodilators. Application of vasodilators is based on the hypotheses that heart failure primarily is a vascular circulatory disease. Vasodilators just as diuretics are hardly new concepts in treating heart failure.

---

[21] Current information on the Cornavita project can be found on the website https://www.cornavita.de/home/

Hence the old saying applies: "If you always do what you've always done, you always get what you've always gotten." No doubt, there is an urgent need for new treatment options that can keep patients out of hospital and treatment costs down.

All available scientific results from ouabain research leave no doubt that this active ingredient has a therapeutic and pharmacological profile that is different not only from Digitalis glycosides but also from other conventional drugs used in heart failure treatment. The therapeutic profile of ouabain with only weakly pronounced inotropy and strong neurohormonal modulation, which manifests itself in vagomimetic stimulation of myocardial metabolism, comes very close to the profile of an ideal heart failure drug.

Ouabain acts on the vegetative nervous system. Its antagonistic components interact with each other in a specific way. Stimulation or inhibition of one always causes a partial stimulation/inhibition of the opponent. This interaction is called "accentuated antagonism". Modulation of the vegetative nervous system that affects both components will therefore always be more effective than the mere blocking of receptors of a component as practiced in conventional therapy with beta blockers and ACE inhibitors.

Ouabain exerts its cardio-protective effects also by activating ouabain-Na/K-ATPase signalosomes, which are independent of the ion pumping function of the sodium pump. These signal cascades induced by ischemic preconditioning as well as by ouabain lead to the protection of almost all internal organs. The effect of the ouabain-NaK-ATPase-signalosomes on the mitochondria important for energy supply explains the clinical experience with ouabain, in which a positive effect on the energy balance of the heart had been observed. While digoxin was known as a "whip for the starving horse" because of its strong inotropy, ouabain was characterized by clinicians as "oats for the starving heart".

The therapeutic effects of ouabain in the treatment of heart failure have been proven in decades of clinical experience. There is no doubt about the effects after intravenous application, they are undisputed. The doubts about reliable effects after oral application are based on ignorance of the importance of galenics, misconceptions about the role of bioavailability and unsuitable indications. The effect is not determined by absolute bioavailability, but by sufficiently high, reproducible concentration in the organism (serum concentration). The mechanisms of action of ouabain, which have been experimentally proven by current research results, prove that this active ingredient has an as yet unexploited potential in the treatment of heart failure. Together with good tolerability, this provides ideal conditions for successful drug development.

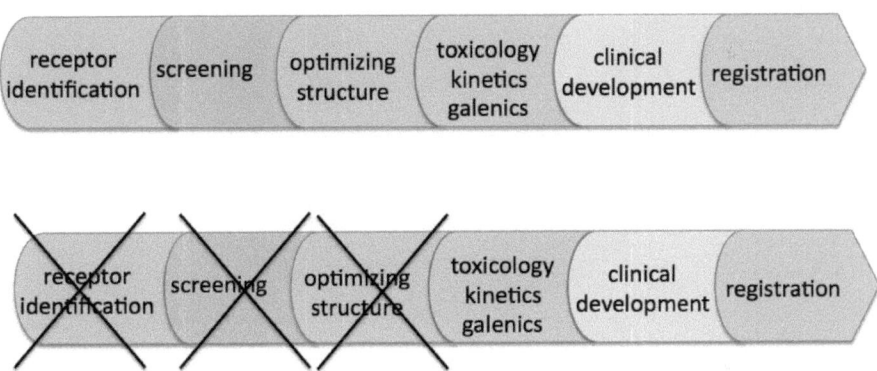

Ouabain belongs chemically to the class of cardiac glycosides, which today are only recommended as reserve drugs in the guidelines for the treatment of chronic heart failure in the form of Digitalis preparations (digoxin, digitoxin). The pharmaceutical industry is no longer interested in these active ingredients. It therefore requires investors willing to take risks and to tap the clinical and economic potential of ouabain.

A comparison of the studies necessary for a new approval of ouabain with the costs for the classical development of a new drug illustrates the relatively low costs required to implement such a project. The active substance, its indications and side effects are known. A large part of the preclinical data is also already available.

Based on a comprehensive analysis of the preclinical and clinical data on uabain described in the scientific literature, the start-up company *Cornavita* is to be founded, which is engaged in the clinical development of this drug in the indication heart failure. A detailed concept is available.

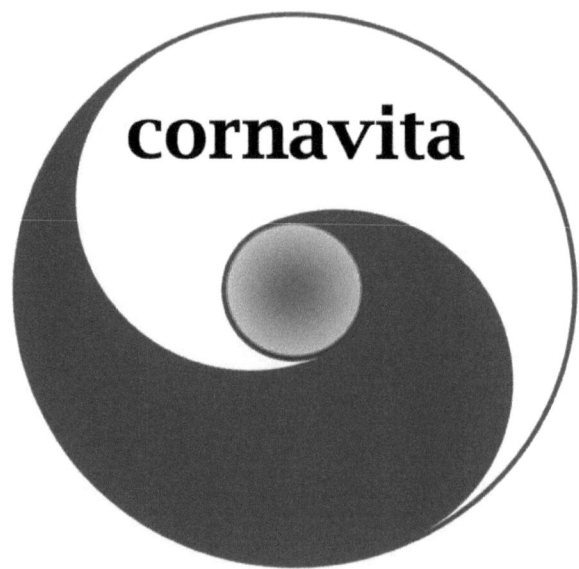

Attractive market potential for heart failure drugs

Heart failure is one of the most common internal diseases. So far, it cannot be treated causally. The main causes of heart failure are coronary heart disease (ischaemic heart disease, angina pectoris), high blood pressure (arterial hypertension) and diseases of the heart muscle. Current treatment strategies for heart failure can improve patients' chances of survival, but they cannot prevent the disease from progressing. All available therapies are limited to symptom relief. Despite modern therapies with beta-blockers, ACE inhibitors and diuretics, the prognosis is still very unfavourable. Overall, half of the patients die within four years. This failure of modern heart failure treatment with beta-blockade and full angiotensin II modulation illustrates the urgent need for better treatments. The interest of clinicians and pharmaceutical companies in substances that offer effective therapy options is correspondingly high. The global market for heart failure drugs is estimated at more than 15 billion US dollars. In the United States alone, more than seven billion US dollars are spent each year on the treatment of heart failure with drugs.

10 years of exclusivity

The active ingredient ouabain and its use in the treatment of heart disease has been known for more than 100 years. Therefore, there are no longer any patents with which an investment in the intended clinical development of ouabain could be secured. Nevertheless, there are sufficient possibilities to guarantee exclusive rights of use and thus comprehensive protection of the investment.

Currently, ouabain is no longer approved worldwide. This results in the possibility of achieving exclusivity and protection of the investment through the regulations laid down in the German Medicines Act. The Medicines Act grants an exclusivity period of 10 years after the approval of the product for all toxicological, pharmacological and clinical data to be prepared for registration. No competitor has access to the submitted documents within this period. Corresponding provisions exist in both European and American regulations. An exclusivity margin of more than ten years is hardly effectively achieved even in the marketing of patented new active ingredients due to the long research and development times.

Cornavita is organised as a project developer

The active ingredient ouabain is commercially available as a pure substance. The formulation development and the preparation of the preclinical data package as well as the clinical development and later on large-scale production of the finished product can be carried out by suitable service providers. Cornavita will organise and manage the entire development process in the form of a tight project management. For each task package - formulation, patents, preclinical, clinical, registration - qualified external experts are involved to ensure sound development.

First stage of development

The clinical effect of ouabain is proven and documented in the literature. For a new approval of ouabain it is nevertheless necessary to create a data package that meets the current requirements of the registration authorities and is suitable to convince clinicians and general practitioners of the efficacy of this drug. This will be done in stages. In the first stage, a suitable galenic dosage form for oral administration is to be developed and its pharmacokinetic and pharmacodynamic profile prepared. An analysis of the doses of different enteral formulations described in the literature shows that it is possible to achieve serum concentrations of ouabain by sublingual application which correspond to those after iv application. In therapeutic practice, iv doses of 0.25 mg - 1.0 mg ouabain per day have proven to be optimal. A steady-state serum concentration of 0.5 ng/ml was measured at this dosage. Based on this, galenic formulations of ouabain are to be optimized to ensure a steady-state serum concentration of 0.5 ng/ml with minimal use of active ingredients.

Second stage of development

As soon as a galenic formulation with this requirement profile is available, the toxicological data required for registration are determined in a second stage and the preclinical data package is completed. Literature data on the acute toxicity of ouabain in various animal species are known. Genotoxicity must be determined. The anti-carcinogenic effect of ouabain found in various animal models suggests that genotoxicity will not cause any problems. Ouabain is not metabolized in the organism, but is excreted unchanged to about two thirds via the kidney and to one third via the intestine. This eliminates the need for own research on metabolism. The required preclinical data package is discussed and defined in detaile with the regulatory authorities.

Third stage of development

The clinical studies to be conducted in a third stage of development are also designed in close cooperation with the registration authorities. Study protocols are defined with an expert panel of recognised cardiologists to ensure that the study results are relevant in practice and meet the requirements of the registration authorities for approval.

Financing of the company

The financing of the company is coordinated with the gradual development. A first financing round will enable the development of an appropriate galenic dosage form and the determination of basic kinetic and pharmacodynamic data.

In a second financing round, sufficient funds will be raised to complete all the data required for clinical trials to begin. A third financing round will then ensure the financing of the pivotal study.

As an alternative to internal financing, discussions with pharmaceutical and biotechnology companies on the joint development of ouabain will begin once the data on the selected galenic dosage form are available.

Only if Cornavita is successful will ouabain, this gift from paradise, be able to enrich the arsenal of drugs for the treatment of heart diseases. Creative approaches to financing must be taken. In addition to the commitment of financially strong partners (VC funds, business angels), the potential of doctors and patients familiar with ouabain must be mobilised. In a fund specially designed for the development of ouabain, smaller sums of interested parties can also be bundled into a sufficient capital stock. A large number of small investors are just as powerful as a financially strong investor. This potential should be used in the interest of affected patients. It is a matter of the heart of this book to encourage all ouabain connoisseurs to participate in the efforts to revive ouabain and to make their active contribution.

$$\approx \quad \approx \approx$$

Please mail suggestions, comments, and notes on the facts and views set down in this book to:

hauke.fuerstenwerth@googlemail.com

References

Ackerknecht EH, Aspects of the History of Therapeutics, Bull History Med **1962**; 36: 389-419

Adams KF Jr, Ghali JK, Herbert Patterson J, Stough WG, Butler J, Bauman JL, Ventura HO, Sabbah H, Mackowiak JI, van Veldhuisen DJ. A perspective on re-evaluating digoxin's role in the current management of patients with chronic systolic heart failure: targeting serum concentration to reduce hospitalization and improve safety profile. Eur J Heart Fail. **2014**; 16(5): 483-493

A. G. Ann Intern Med **1951**, S. 1390

Agostini PG, Doria E, Berti M, Guazzi MD, Lomg-term use of k-Strophanthin in advanced congestive heart failure due to dilated cardiomyopathy: A double-blind crossover evaluation versus digoxin. Clin Cardiol **1994**; 17: 536 – 541

Altmann K, Zur lingualen Strophanthin Resorption auf Grund klinischer und experimenteller Ergebnisse, Hippokrates. **1952**; 23(15): 417-419.

Altmann K, (1952 b) Beitrag zur peroralen Strophanthintherapie. Med Klin (Munich). **1952**; 47(14): 446-448.

Ambrosy AP, Butler J, Ahmed A, Vaduganathan M, van Veldhuisen DJ, Colucci WS, Gheorghiade M. The use of digoxin in patients with worsening chronic heart failure: reconsidering an old drug to reduce hospital admissions. J Am Coll Cardiol. **2014**; 63(18): 1823-1832

Amgen Inc. Pressemitteilung vom 21. Juli **2015**

Ardenne M, Reitnauer P G, Messungen zu Elementarvorgängen des Herzinfarktes. Card. Bull. Acta Cardiol **1971**; 4/5: 51 – 72

Ardenne M, Kern B, „Der Herzinfarkt als Folge der lysomalen Zytolyse Kettenreaktion", Dtsch. Ges.wesen, **1971**; 26: 1769 – 1780

Ardenne M ; Reitnauer P G ; Rohde K, Zum pH-Verhalten des Myokards und seiner Bedeutung für Herzinfarkt- und Krebs-Mehrschritt-Therapie. Wien Klin Wochenschr, **1972**; 84 (3): 47–54

Ardenne M, Die Hemmung der Mikrozirkulation beim Myokardinfardt und das perlingual applizierte g-Strophanthin. Neue Vorstellungen zum Mechanismus des Myokardinfarktes und seiner Bekämpfung. Arzneimittel-Forschung **1978**; 28(12): 2315–2326

Aschenbrenner R, Foth K. Wiederbelebung der oralen Strophanthin-Therapie? Dtsch Med Wochenschr. **1951** Aug 31;76(35):1057-61.

Aschenbrenner R, Foth K. Herzglykoside und Antikoagulantien in der Therapie des frischen Myocardinfarkts. Med Klin (Munich). **1956**; 51(17): 716-723.

Baecher S, Kroiss M, Fassnacht M, Vogeser M. No endogenous ouabain is detectable in human plasma by ultra-sensitive UPLC-MS/MS. Clin Chim Acta. **2014**; 431: 87–92.

Baker PF, Blaustein MP, Hodgkin AL, Steinhardt RA. The influence of calcium on sodium efflux in squid axons. J Physiol. **1969**; 200(2): 431-58.

Belz GG, Matthews J, Sauer U, Stern H, Schneider B. Pharmacodynamic effects of Ouabain following single sublingual and intravenous doses in normal subjects. Eur J clin Pharmacol, **1984**; 26: 187 – 292

Berghaus A, Winau R, *Probleme der Standardisierung von Digitalispräparaten*, in Neue Beiträge zur Arzneimittelgeschichte, Veröffentlichungen der Internationalen Gesellschaft für Geschichte der Pharmazie e.V. Band 51, **1982**

Blaustein MP, Livin' with NCX and lovin' it: a 45 year romance. Adv Exp Med Biol. **2013**; 961: 3-15.

Blaustein MP, Why isn't endogenous ouabain more widely accepted? Am J Physiol Heart Circ Physiol. **2014**;3 07: 635–639

Blaustein MP, The pump, the exchanger, and the holy spirit: origins and 40-year evolution of ideas about the ouabain-Na+ pump endocrine system. Am J Physiol Cell Physiol. **2018** Jan 1;314(1):C3-C26.

Bonah C, Albert Fraenkel, die Medizinische Fakultät Strassburg und die Entstehung der der Strophanthintherapie, in Drings P, Thierfelder J, Weidmann B., Willig F., Albert Fraenkel. Ein Arztleben in Licht und Schatten, 1864- 1938, Ecomed, Landsberg, **2004**, pp. 155-186.

Bonah, C, "We need for digitalis preparations what the state has established for serum therapy ... " From collecting plants to international standardization: the Strophanthin case, 1900-1938, in Christoph Gradmann and

Jonathan Simon, Evaluating and Standardizing Therapeutic Agents 1890-1950, London, Palgrave, **2010**, pp. 202-228.

Boros J, Strophoral: Ein therapeutischer Irrtum. Münchener medizinische Wochenschrift **1951**; 93 (20): 1026–1030

Bretschneider H J, Frank A ; Kanzow E, Bernard U, Über das Verhalten der Milchsäureausnutzung des Koronarblutes zur venösen Sauerstoffsättigung. Verh Dtsch Ges Kreislaufforsch, **1956**; 22: 300–305

Buckalew VM, Endogenous digitalis-like factors: An overview of the history. Front. Endocrinol., **2015**; 6: 49
http://journal.frontiersin.org/article/10.3389/fendo.2015.00049/full

Burger, Wenzel, Erfahrungen mit der perlingualen Strophanthin-Therapie., Ärztl. Praxis V/30 (**1953**)

Buzaglo N, Golomb M, Rosen H, Beeri R, Ami HC, Langane F, Pierre S, Lichtstein D, Augmentation of Ouabain-Induced Increase in Heart Muscle Contractility by Akt Inhibitor MK-2206. J Cardiovasc Pharmacol Ther. **2018** Jan 1:1074248418788301.

Candilio L, Malik A, Hausenloy DJ. Protection of organs other than the heart by remote ischemic conditioning. J Cardiovasc Med (Hagerstown). **2013**; 14: 193 – 205.

Chasalow F, Pierce-Cohen L. Ionotropin is the mammalian digoxin-like material (DLM). It is a phosphocholine ester of a steroid with 23 carbon atoms. Steroids. 2018 Aug;136:63-75.

Christophersen H, Der Schlüssel zur Infarktverhütung, Kindler Verlag GmbH, München, **1973**, S. 113

Cole GD, Francis DP. Trials are best, ignore the rest: safety and efficacy of digoxin. BMJ **2015**; 351: H4662. DOI: 10.1136/BMJ.H4662

Cotter G, Cohen-Solal A, Davison BA, Mebazaa A. RELAX-AHF, BLAST-AHF, TRUE-AHF, and other important truths in acute heart failure research. Eur J Heart Fail **2017**;19:1355–7.

Curschmann H, Jores A, Lehrbuch der speziellen Therapie innerer Krankheiten, Springer Verlag **1947**

Curschmann H, Über unsinnige Therapie, Med Klin. **1947**; 42(1): 25–27 de Boer A, Cohen AF. Digoxin and mortality: lessons for observational studies. Br J Clin Pharmacol. **2015** Sep 22. doi: 10.1111/bcp.12791.

Dietz E, Albert Fraenkel, C. F. Boehringer & Söhne und die intravenöse Strophanthintherapie in Peter Drings, Jörg Thierfelder, Bernd Weidemann, Friedrich Willig (Hrsg.), Michael Ehmann (Mitarbeit): Albert Fraenkel – Ein Arztleben in Licht und Schatten 1864–1938. Verlag Ecomed, Landsberg **2004**.

Edens E, Die Strophanthinbehandlung der Angina pectoris, Münchner medizinische Wochenschrift **1934**; 37: 1424-1427

Edens E, Digitalisfibel für den Arzt, fünfte Auflage, Springer Verlag, **1944**

Edens E, Die Digitalisbehandlung, Verlag Urban & Schwarzenberg, Berlin-München **1948**Eichholtz F, Lehrbuch der Pharmakologie, Springer Verlag, **1947**

E. Merck, Digitalis-Glykoside und verwandte Arzneistoffe, E. Merck's wissenschaftliche Abhandlungen aus den Gebieten der Pharmakotherapie, Pharmazie und verwandter Disziplinen Nr. 8, 2. umgearbeitete Auflage **1914**, available online at the Digitale Bibliothek Braunschweig http://www.digibib.tu-bs.de/?docid=00037515. This paper contains an overview of the large number of cardiac glycoside preparations known at that time.

Erdle HP, Schultz KD, Wetzel E, Gross F. Resorption und Ausscheidung von g-Strophanthin nach intravenöser und perlingualer Gabe. Dtsch Med Wochenschr. **1979**; 104(27): 976-979.

Erdmann E, Über die Therapie mit oralem und intravenösem Strophanthin, in: An den Grenzen der Schulmedizin, hrsg. von Irmgard Oepen, Deutscher Ärzte Verlag, Köln, **1985**

Forth W, Furukawa E, Rummel W. Vergleichende Untersuchung von Resorption und Ausscheidung tritium-markierter Herzglykoside. Naunyn Schmiedebergs Arch Exp Pathol Pharmakol. **1969**; 262(1): 53-72.

Franck R, Moderne Therapie in innerer Medizin und Allgemeinpraxis, Springer Verlag, Berlin **1943**

Fraenkel A, Über die physiologische Dosierung von Digitalispräparaten, Therapie der Gegenwart **1902**; 43:106-112

Fraenkel A, Zur Digitalistherapie. Über intravenöse Strophanthintherapie, Verh Kongr Inn Med **1906**, 257-265

Fraenkel A, Abhandlungen zur Digitalistherapie. Über intravenöse Strophanthininjektionen bei Herzkranken, Naunyn-Schmiedeberg's Archives of Pharmacology **1907**; 57(1/2): 79-122

Fraenkel A, Abhandlungen zur Digitalistherapie. III. Bemerkungen zur internen Digitalismedikation. Naunyn-Schmiedeberg's Archives of Pharmacology **1907**; 57(1/2): 131-136

Fraenkel A, Schwartz G, Über Digitaliswirkung an gesunden und an kompensierten Herzkranken, Archiv für experimentelle Pathologie und Pharmakologie, Supplementband **1908**, Festschrift Oswald Schmiedeberg S. 188-198

Fraenkel A, Strophanthin Therapie, Verlag Julius von Springer, Berlin **1933**

Fraenkel A, Von der empirischen zur experimentellen Digitalistherapie, Schweizerische Medizinische Wochenschrift **1936**;18:434 - 440

Fürstenwerth H, Ouabain and endogenous ouabain - Dr. Jekyll and Mr. Hyde of cardiac glycosides? British Journal of Medicine and Medical Research, **2015**; 8(5): 477-484

Gable ME, Ellis L, Fedorova OV, Bagrov AY, Askari A, Comparison of Digitalis sensitivities of Na/K-ATPases from human and pig kidneys, ACS Omega **2017**, 2, 3610-3615

Garbe A, Nowak H. Zur Pharmakokinetik des Pruvosid. Arzneimittelforschung. **1968**; 18(12): 1597-601.

Gheorghiade M, Hall VB, Jacobsen G, Alam M, Rosman H, Goldstein S. Effects of increasing maintenance dose of digoxin on left ventricular function and neurohormones in patients with chronic heart failure treated with diuretics and angiotensin-converting enzyme inhibitors. Circulation. **1995**; 92: 1801–1807

Ghirardi P, Marzo A, Gianfranceschi M, Bertoli L, Conti F, Mantero O. Plasma levels and urinary excretion of K-strophanthoside (3H) administered rectally to human subjects. Arzneimittelforschung. **1973** Nov;23(11):1547-50.

Gilg, Thoms, Schedel: Die Strophanthinfrage. Berlin **1904**.

Gillis RA. Cardiac sympathetic nerve activity: Changes induced by ouabain and propranolol. Science. **1969**; 166(3904): 508-510.

Gillis RA. Digitalis: A neuroexcitatory drug. Circulation. **1975**; 52: 739-742.

Gillmann H, Stellungnahme zur peroralen Strophanthinprophylaxe des Herzinfarktes, Deutsches Ärzteblatt, **1971**; 44: 2929 - 2936

Godfraind T, Stimulation and inhibition of the Na+/K+-pump by cardiac glycosides, In: Erdmann E, Greeff K, Skou JC, editors. Cardiac glycosides 1785–1985. New York: Springer Verlag; **1986**, p 381 – 393

Gonder U, Worm N. Mehr Fett: Liebeserklärung an einen zu Unrecht verteufelten Nährstoff. Systemed Verlag GmbH, **2010**

Graham RM, Frazier DP, Thompson JW, Haliko S, Li H, Wasserlauf BJ, Spiga MG, Bishopric NH, Webster KA. A unique pathway of cardiac myocyte death caused by hypoxia-acidosis. J Exp Biol. **2004**; 207(Pt 18): 3189-3200.

Granger CB, McMurray JJ. Using measures of disease progression to determine therapeutic effect: a sirens' song. J Am Coll Cardiol. **2006**; 48(3): 434-437

Greeff K, Köhler E, Strobach H, Verspohl E. Zur Pharmakokinetik des g-Strophanthins, Verh Dtsch Ges Kreislaufforsch. **1974**; 40: 301-305

Greef K Schadewaldt H *Introduction and Remarks on the History of Cardiac Glycosides,* in Cardiac Glycosides part I, Hrsg Greef K, Springer Verlag Berlin Heidelberg New York **1981**

Greene J A, Prescribing by the numbers, drugs and the definition of disease, The John Hopkins University Press, **2007**

Gremels H. Die vegetative-hormonale Stoffwechselsteuerung und ihre Bedeutung für die Pharmakologie. Klin Wochenschr. 1946-1947;24-25(29-30):449-453.

Haasis, R, Digitalisglykoside und EKG, perimed Fachbuch-Verlagsgesellschaft, Erlangen, **1983**

Halhuber M, Lantscherat T, Meusburger K. Zur Strophoraltherapie. Med Klin. **1954**;36:1440-1443

Hamlyn JM, Blaustein MP, Bova S, DuCharme DW, Harris DW, Mandel F, Mathews WR, Ludens JH. Identification and characterization of a ouabain-like compound from human plasma. Proc Natl Acad Sci U S A. **1991**; 88: 6259–6263.

Healey CM, Kumbhani DJ, Healey NA et al. Impact of intraoperative myocardial tissue acidosis on postoperative adverse outcomes and cost of care for patients undergoing prolonged aortic clamping during cardiopulmonary bypass. Am J Surg **2009**; 197: 203–210

Heilmeyer L, Bemerkungen zum Strophoralstreit, Münch Med Wochenschr. **1952** Feb 1;94(5):208-209

Herrmann, Die Wirksamkeit oraler Strophanthintherapie, Der Deutsche Apotheker, **1999**; 42(4): 113 - 116

Hochrein H. Electrolytes in heart failure and myocardial hypoxia. Vasc Dis. **1966**; 3(3): 196-200.

Hokkanen M, Imperial Networks, Colonial Bioprospecting and Bur-roughs Wellcome & Co.: The Case of Strophanthus Kombe from Ma-lawi (1859–1915), Social History of Medicine **2012**; 25(3): 589–607

Ingwall JS, Weiss RG. Is the failing heart energy starved? On using chemical energy to support cardiac function. Circ Res. **2004**;95(2):135-145.

Ingwall JS, Energy metabolism in heart failure and remodelling. Cardiovascular Research **2009**; 81: 412–419

Kharbanda RK1, Nielsen TT, Redington AN, Translation of remote ischaemic preconditioning into clinical practice. Lancet. **2009**; 374(9700): 1557-65.

Kingdon J, Agwanda B, Kinnaird M, O'Brien T, Holland C, Gheysens T, Boulet-Audet M, Vollrath F. A poisonous surprise under the coat of the African crested rat. Proc Biol Sci. **2012**;279(1729):675-80.

Kern B, Grundlagen der Inneren Medizin, Ferdinand Enke Verlag, Stuttgart, **1946**

Kern B, Die Herzinsuffizienz, Ferdinand Enke Verlag, Stuttgart, **1948**

Kern B, Strophoral - Zur Erneuerung der oralen Strophanthustherapie Dtsch med Wochenschr **1949**; 74(33/34): 1017-1021

Kern B, Die orale Strophanthin-Behandlung, Ferdinand Enke Verlag, Stuttgart, **1951**

Kern B, Zum Nachweis der Strophanthin-Resorption. Medizinische Monatsschrift, **1952**; 6, (6): 371–374

Kern B, Der Myokardinfarkt, 3. Auflage, Haug Verlag, **1974**

Kesselheim AS, Avorn J, The most transformative drugs of the past 25 years: a survey of physicians, Nat Rev Drug Discov. **2013**; 12(6): 425-431

Khodus GR, Kruusmägi M, Li J, Liu XL, Aperia A. Calcium signaling triggered by ouabain protects the embryonic kidney from adverse developmental programming. Pediatr Nephrol. **2011**; 26(9): 1479-82.

Kotsovsky D, Therapie des Altersherz, Ärztl. Praxis V/6 (**1953**)

Kottmann K., Zeitschrift für klinische Medizin, **1905,** Bd. H2, 56

Krämer, K.-D, Ghabussi, P, Hochrein H, Klinische Untersuchungen über die orale und parenterale Wirksamkeit von k-Strophanthin-α an dekompensierten Herzkranken. Deutsche Medizinische Wochenschrift – DMW **1972**; 97; 22: 870–875

Krause D. Förderung und Sicherung der enteralen Resorption von G-Strophanthin durch Natriumlaurylsulfat. Arzneimittelforschung. **1955**; 5(8): 428-432.

Lampe K, Ein Beitrag zur oralen Strophanthintherapie. Med Welt. **1968**; 26: 1569-72.

Laugsand LE, Strand LB, Platou C, Vatten LJ, Janszky, Insomnia and the risk of incident heart failure: a population study. Eur Heart J. **2014**; 35(21): 1382-1393.

Leuenberger H, Gesund durch Gift, Deutsche Verlagsanstalt Stuttgart, **1972**

Leuschner, Toxicological studies with Ouabain, Naunyn Schmiedebergs Arch Pharmacol. **2001**; 363 (4) suppl, 139, abstract 544

Lewis LK, Yandle TG, Hilton PJ, Jensen BP, Begg EJ, and Nicholls MG. Endogenous Ouabain Is Not Ouabain. Hypertension. **2014**; 64(4): 680-3

Li J, Khodus GR, Kruusmagi M, Kamali-Zare P, Liu XL, Eklof AC, Zelenin S, Brismar H, Aperia A, Ouabain protects against adverse developmental programming of the kidney. Nat Commun. **2010**; 27; 1:42.

Lindenbaum J, Mellow MH, Blackstone MO, Butler VP Jr. Variation in biologic availability of digoxin from four preparations. N Engl J Med. **1971**; 285(24): 1344-1347.

Liu J, Tian J, Haas M, et al. Ouabain interaction with cardiac Na/K-ATPase initiates signal cascades independent of changes in intracellular Na+ and Ca2+ concentrations. J Biol Chem **2000**; 275:27838–27844

Liu L, Wu J, Kennedy DJ, Regulation of Cardiac Remodeling by Cardiac Na(+)/K(+)-ATPase Isoforms. Front Physiol. 2016; 7: 382. doi: 10.3389/fphys.2016.00382. eCollection **2016**

Lüllmann H, Peters T, Preuner J. Mechanism of action of digitalis glycosides in the light of new experimental observations. Eur Heart J **1982**; 3 Suppl D: 45-51.

Lüllmann H, Peters T, Prillwitz HH, et al. Cardiac glycosides with different effects in the heart. Basic Res Cardiol **1984**;7 9 Suppl: 93-101.

Marzilli M, Merz CN, Boden WE, Bonow RO, Capozza PG, Chilian WM, DeMaria AN, Guarini G, Huqi A, Morrone D, Patel MR, Weintraub WS. Obstructive coronary atherosclerosis and ischemic heart disease: an elusive link! J Am Coll Cardiol. **2012**; 60(11)951-956

Marzouk SA, Buck RP, Dunlap LA, Johnson TA, Cascio WE. Measurement of extracellular pH, K(+), and lactate in ischemic heart. Anal Biochem. **2002**; 308(1): 52-60.

Maehder K. Über den Nachweis der perlingualen Strophanthin-Resorption mittels Isotopen. Med Klin (Munich), **1955**; 50(2): 104-5.

Marchetti GV, Marzo A, De Ponti C, Scalvini A, Merlo L, Noseda V. Blood levels and tissue distribution of 3 H-ouabain administered per os. An experimental and clinical study. Arzneimittelforschung. **1971**; 21(9): 1399-403.

Marck PV, Pierre SV. Na/K-ATPase Signaling and Cardiac Pre/Postconditioning with Cardiotonic Steroids. Int J Mol Sci. **2018** Aug 9;19(8). pii: E2336.

Mebazaa A, Acute Heart Failure Deserves a Log-Scale Boost in Research Support: Call for Multidisciplinary and Universal Actions. JACC Heart Fail. **2018** Jan;6(1):76-79.

McMichael J. Pharmacology of the failing human heart. Br Med J. 1948;2(4586):927- 933.

Medscape, Steve Stiles, After Sinking in, PARADIGM-HF Critiqued at HFSA Sessions, September 25, **2014**, http://www.medscape.com/viewarticle/832290#vp_1

Mutschler P, Zur Verbesserung der oralen Strophanthintherapie. Medizinische Klinik (Munich) **1952**; 47(50): 1656–1657

Niedner R, Taschenbuch der Digitalis-Therapie, Georg Thieme Verlag, Stuttgart, **1961**

NEJM Journal watch, Vinay Prasad, Let's Take a Close Look at PARADIGM-HF, September 1, **2014**, http://blogs.jwatch.org/cardioexchange/2014/09/01/lets-scrutinize-paradigm-hf/

Nesher M, Shpolansky U, Viola N, Dvela M, Buzaglo N, Cohen Ben-Ami H, Rosen H, Lichtstein D. Ouabain attenuates cardiotoxicity induced by other cardiac steroids. Br J Pharmacol. **2010** May;160(2):346-54.

Newton GE, Tong JH, Schofield AM, Baines AD, Floras JS, Parker JD. Digoxin reduces cardiac sympathetic activity in severe congestive heart failure. J Am Coll Cardiol. **1996**; 28: 155–161.

Okita GT. Dissociation of Na+,K+-ATPase inhibition from digitalis inotropy. Fed Proc **1977**; 36(9): 2225-2233

Olfson M, Marcus S C, Decline In Placebo-Controlled Trial Results Suggests New Directions For Comparative Effectiveness Research, Health Aff, June **2013**; 32: 1116-1125

Popper K, Logik der Forschung: zur Erkenntnistheorie der modernen Naturwissenschaften, Springer Verlag Wien, **1935**

Osseo-Asare, Bitter roots: the search for healing plants in Africa, The University of Chicago Press, **2014**

Packer M, Acute Heart Failure Is an Event Rather Than a Disease: Plea for a Radical Change in Thinking and in Therapeutic Drug Development. JACC Heart Fail. **2018** Jan;6(1):73-75.

Prescrire , New drugs and indications in 2010: inadequate assessment; patients at risk, Rev Prescrire February **2011**; 31 (328): 134-141

Raab W, Clinical course of 200 cases of angina pectoris treated with roentgen irradiation of the adrenals (1937-1947). Am J Roentgenol Radium Ther. **1950**; 63(6): 895-901

Raab W, Chaplin JP, Bajusz E. Myocardial necroses produced in domesticated rats and in wild rats by sensory and emotional stresses. Proc Soc Exp Biol Med. **1964**; 116: 665-669

Raab W, Über 45 Jahre Arzt, Therapie der Gegenwart, **1966**; 105(2): 224-230

Raab W. Koronarinsuffiozienz, Katecholamine, Kortikoide und Kalium. Wien Klin Wochenschr. **1966**; 78(41): 684-7.

Reindell, H, Weyland, R, Bilger, R, Klepzig, H. Zur Frage der Resorbierbarkeit des herzwirksamen Glykosids im Strophoral. Munch Med Wochenschr. **1952**; 94(6): 266–273

Robergs, R. A., Ghiasvand, F, Parker D, Biochemistry of exercise-induced metabolic acidosis. Am. J. Physiol. Regul. Integr. Comp. Physiol. **2004**; 287: 502-516.

Roth K, Nachweis der Herzwirkung von Purostrophan-Dragées. Ther Ggw. **1955**; 94(8): 292-295.

Ruiz-Torres A. Kinetik der Herzglykoside im Organismus des Menschen und der Versuchstiere. Klin Wochenschr. **1970**; 48(5): 257-70.

Runge TM, Stephens JC, Holden P, Havemann DF, Kilgore WM, Dale EM, Dalton RE. Pharmacodynamic distinctions between ouabain, digoxin and digitoxin. Arch Int Pharmacodyn Ther. **1975**; 214(1): 31-45.

Runge TM, Clinical implications of differences in pharmacodynamic action of polar and nonpolar cardiac glycosides. Am Heart J. **1977**; 93(2):248-55.

Salz H, Schneider B, Perlinguales g-Strophanthin bei stabiler Angina pectoris, Zeitschrift für Allgemeinmedizin **1985**; 61: 1223 -1228

Sarre H, Indikation der verschiedenen Herzglykoside bei ambulanter Behandlung von Herzkranken. Die Medizinische Welt **1951**; 20(35-36): 1065–1070

Sarre H, Strophanthinbehandlung bei Angina pectoris. Therapiewoche **1952/53**; 3: 311-314

Schaefer H, Herzinfarkt - Vorspann. In Schaefer, Jentsch, Huber, Wegener: Herzinfarkt Report 2000, Verlag Urban&Fischer, München, **2000**

Schedel, Die Strophanthus-Frage vom pharmakologischen und klinischen Standpunkt, Berichte der Deutschen Pharmakologischen Gesellschaft, **1904**, S. 120 ff

Schettler G, Weber E, Kübler W, Orales Strophanthin in der Therapie der Herzkrankheiten und speziell der koronaren Herzkrankheiten, Deutsches Ärzteblatt **1977**; 15: 995 - 998

Schimert G. Klinische Symptomatologie der Herzinsuffizienz und der funktionellen Herzschwäche. Arztl Forsch. **1967**; 21(3): 104-12.

Schmidsberger P, Skandal Herzinfarkt, Verlag R.S. Schulz **1975**

Seiler C. Collateral Circulation of the Heart. London, UK: Springer-Verlag; **2009**.

Seiler C, Meier P. Historical aspects and relevance of the human coronary collateral circulation. Curr Cardiol Rev. **2014**; 10(1): 2-16.

Selye H, The pluricausal cardiopathies, Verlag C.C. Thomas, Springfield, **1961**

Silva E, Soares-da-Silva P. New Insights into the Regulation of Na(+),K(+)-ATPase by Ouabain. Int Rev Cell Mol Biol. **2012**; 294: 99-132

Silva PA, Monnerat-Cahli G, Pereira-Acácio A, Luzardo R, Sampaio LS, Luna-Leite MA, Lara LS, Einicker-Lamas M, Panizzutti R, Madeira C, Vieira-Filho LD, Castro-Chaves C, Ribeiro VS, Paixão AD, Medei E, Vieyra A. Mechanisms Involving Ang II and MAPK/ERK1/2 Signaling Pathways Underlie Cardiac and Renal Alterations during Chronic Undernutrition. PLoS One. **2014**; 9(7): e100410.

Simonini M, Casanova P, Citterio L, Messaggio E, Lanzani C, Manunta P. Endogenous Ouabain and Related Genes in the Translation from Hypertension to Renal Diseases. Int J Mol Sci. **2018** Jul 3;19(7). pii: E1948.

Skou J. C. William Withering – The man and his work, in Cardiac Glycosides 1785 – 1985, Hrsg E. Erdmann, K. Greef, J. C. Skou, Steinkopf Verlag, Darmstadt **1986**

Somberg J, Greenfield B, Tepper D, Digitalis: Historical Development in Clinical Medicine, J Clin Pharmacol **1985**;25: 484 – 489

SPIEGEL, Hungernde Herzen, 19. 11. **1971**
http://www.spiegel.de/spiegel/print/d-44914474.html

SPIEGEL, Burda's biedere Bunte, 9. 9. **1964**,
http://www.spiegel.de/spiegel/print/d-46175278.html

Staessen JA, Thijs L, Stolarz-Skrzypek K, et al. Main results of the ouabain and adducin for Specific Intervention on Sodium in Hypertension Trial (OASIS-HT): a randomized placebo-controlled phase-2 dose-finding study of rostafuroxin. Trials. **2011**;12:13

Strobach H, Wirth KE, Rojsathaporn K. Absorption, metabolism and elimination of strophanthus glycosides in man. Naunyn Schmiedebergs Arch Pharmacol. **1986**; 334(4): 496-500.

Taegtmeyer H, McNulty P, Young ME. Adaptation and maladaptation of the heart in diabetes: Part I: general concepts. Circulation. **2002** ;105(14): 1727-1733.

Teicholz N. The Big Fat Surprise: Why Butter, Meat and Cheese Belong in a Healthy Diet. Simon & Schuster; Reprint edition, **2015**

The SPRINT Research Group, A Randomized Trial of Intensive versus Standard Blood-Pressure Control. N Engl J Med. **2015** Nov 9. [Epub ahead of print] DOI: 10.1056/NEJMoa1511939

Tijmstra T, The psychological and social implicationsof serum cholesterolscreening, International Journal of Risk and Safety in Medicine **1990**; 1: 29-44

van Bilsen M, Patel HC, Bauersachs J, Böhm M, Borggrefe M, Brutsaert D, Coats AJS, de Boer RA, de Keulenaer GW, Filippatos GS, Floras J, Grassi G, Jankowska EA, Kornet L, Lunde IG, Maack C, Mahfoud F, Pollesello P, Ponikowski P, Ruschitzka F, Sabbah HN, Schultz HD, Seferovic P, Slart RHJA, Taggart P, Tocchetti CG, Van Laake LW, Zannad F, Heymans S, Lyon AR. The autonomic nervous system as a therapeutic target in heart failure: a scientific position statement from the Translational Research Committee of the Heart Failure Association of the European Society of Cardiology. Eur J Heart Fail. **2017** Nov;19(11):1361-1378.

Vaquez H, Ouabaine. Arch. Mal. Coeur **1917**; 10: 467

Venugopal J, Blanco G, On the Many Actions of Ouabain: Pro-Cystogenic Effects in Autosomal Dominant Polycystic Kidney Disease. Molecules. **2017** May 3; 22(5): E729.

Wasserstrom JA, Farkas DE. Inotropic and toxic actions of several cardiac steroids in sheep cardiac tissues. Prog Clin Biol Res **1988**; 268B: 469–476.

Wasserstrom JA, Farkas DE, Norell MA, et al. Effects of different cardiac steroids on intracellular sodium, inotropy and toxicity in sheep Purkinje fibers. J Pharmacol Exp Ther **1991**; 258: 918–925.

Wasserstrom JA, Aistrup GL. Digitalis: new actions for an old drug. Am J Physiol Heart Circ Physiol **2005**; 289: 1781-1793

Weber, J Die perorale Strophanthintherapie. Medizinische Klinik (Munich) **1955**; 50 (13): 533–535

Wechter WJ, Benaksas EJ. Natriuretic hormones. Prog Drug Res (**1990**) 34:231–60

WHO, Interim Summary of Conclusions and Dietary Recommendations on Total Fat & Fatty Acids. From the Joint FAO/WHO Expert Consultation on Fats and Fatty Acids in Human Nutrition, 10-14 November, **2008**, Geneva http://www.who.int/nutrition/topics/FFA_summary_rec_conclusion.pdf

Wiesend W, Über perorale Strophanthinbehandlung, besonders beim Altersherz. Münchener medizinische Wochenschrift, **1956**; 98(26): 900–904

Wiesend W, Über theoretisch-experimentelle und klinische Grundlagen der peroralen Strophanthinbehandlung. Therapeutische Umschau. Revue thérapeutique, **1956**; 13(9): 172–176 [Wiesend **1956-b**]

Windt R, Boeschen D, Glaeske G, Zentrum für Sozialpolitik – Universität Bremen, Innovationsreport **2013**, Auswertungsergebnisse von Routinedaten der Techniker Krankenkasse aus den Jahren 2010 und 2011

Wu J, Li D, Du L, Baldawi M, Gable ME, Askari A, Liu L. Ouabain prevents pathological cardiac hypertrophy and heart failure through activation of phosphoinositide 3-kinase α in mouse. Cell Biosci. **2015** Nov 18;5:64.

ZEIT, Die „Bunte" treibts zu bunt, 14. 8. **1964**, http://www.zeit.de/1964/33/die-bunte-treibts-zu-bunt/komplettansicht

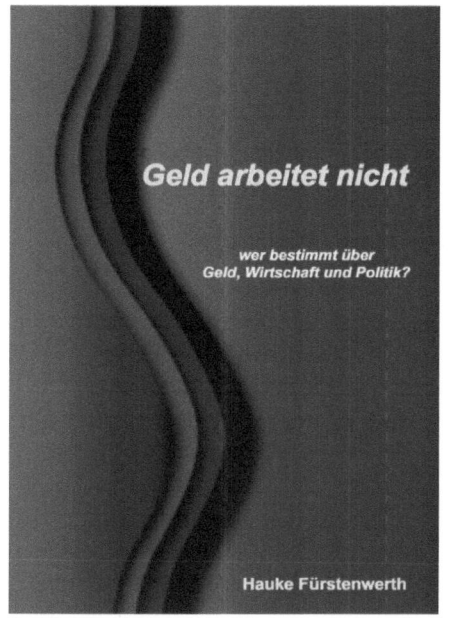

Hauke Fürstenwerth
Geld arbeitet nicht
- wer bestimmt über Geld,
Wirtschaft und Politik?

Shaker Media,
Dezember 2007
ISBN 978-3-940459-22-0
330 Seiten,
16 cm x 23 cm, 24,80 EUR

Die Finanzwirtschaft dominiert über die Realwirtschaft. Geldverwalter diktieren der Gesellschaft und der Politik ihre eigenen Regeln. Ihr Antrieb ist Gier. Gier ist tief im Wesen der Menschen verankert. In der Anonymität der Handelsräume an den Börsen gibt es keine Skrupel oder moralische Abwägungen. Hier wird maßlose Gier hemmungslos ausgelebt. Es herrscht Verteilungskampf. Der Zeitgeist drängt darauf, dieses Prinzip auf die Realwirtschaft zu übertragen. Die Grundlage jedes Wirtschaftens - Mehrwert schaffen - wird damit zerstört.

Hauke Fürstenwerth illustriert an Hand von Fakten das Geschehen in der Finanzwirtschaft. Er zeigt an konkreten Beispielen wie Geld verwaltet wird, wie Hedgefonds, Private-Equity-Fonds und Venture Capital Fonds arbeiten. Er identi ziert die Hauptursachen für die wirtschaftlichen Probleme unserer Zeit: die Gier der Finanzmanager, deren ideologische Rechtfertigung durch den Neoliberalismus und dessen Umsetzung in praktische Politik. Diese Kombination verlagert das Gewinnstreben von der Realwirtschaft in die Finanzwirtschaft. Sie führt damit zur schleichenden Erosion der Sozialen Marktwirtschaft.

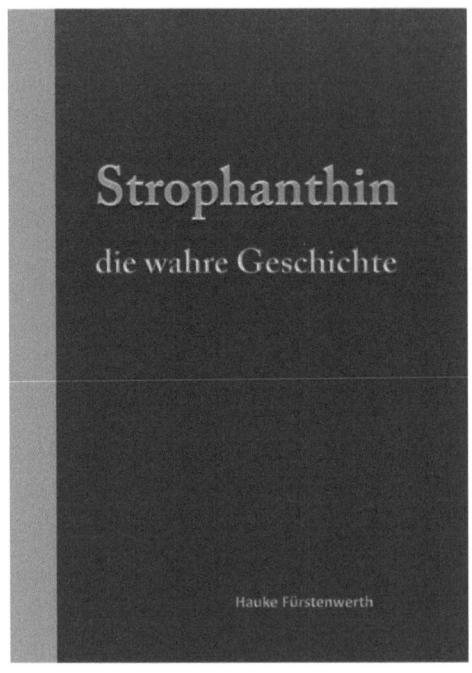

Hauke Fürstenwerth
Strophanthin
die wahre Geschichte

Books on Demand,
Februar 2016
ISBN 978-3739213521
236 Seiten,
15 cm x 21 cm, 22,50 EUR

Strophanthin ist ein Herzmedikament. Es gehört zur Klasse der herzaktiven Steroidglykoside und wird wie diese aus Pflanzen gewonnen. Bis in die 1980er Jahre hinein ist es in Deutschland zur Behandlung von Herzinsuffizienz eingesetzt worden. Wie kaum ein anderes Medikament hat Strophanthin die Zunft der Ärzte in Deutschland polarisiert. Von Befürwortern wurde es als Insulin des Herzens gefeiert, von Gegnern als Placebo verunglimpft. Euphorisches Lob und vernichtende Kritik prägten einen überaus polemisch und emotional geführten Streit zwischen praktischen Ärzten und Hochschulklinikern.

 Das Buch schildert Aufstieg und Fall des Strophanthins. Hauke Fürstenwerth präsentiert eine objektive, an belegbaren Fakten orientierte Aufarbeitung der wahren Geschichte des Strophanthins. Mit bisher nicht bekannten Tatsachen schildert er die wechselvolle Geschichte dieses Arzneimittels. Strophanthin verfügt über ein nicht ausgeschöpftes therapeutisches Potenzial. Das Buch zeigt auf, wie Strophanthin zum Nutzen von Herzpatienten wieder zugelassen werden kann.